praise for e

Every 21 seconds is the most honest book written by a TBI survivor that I have ever read. I am the mother of a 25-year old daughter who suffered the devastating effects of a traumatic brain injury three years ago and I believe I have read almost all of the books written on this topic.

"As a person who is twenty-seven years post brain injury, Every 21 Seconds was a great read and, on some pages, a trip down memory lane for me. It is a poignant book that delves into a world that many know but few understand. It is my hope that it will help educate people about traumatic brain injury and its many ups and downs. It is a book that all of corporate America should be required to read, as well as many medical professionals. The road through brain injury recovery has many twists and turns for everyone. It isn't a one-person disability but a whole-family disability. Brian's triumphant story is an unbelievable accomplishment. I am so proud of him."

–Marvel Vena, past president of the Brain Injury Association of Illinois, a founding member of the Governor's Brain and Spinal Cord Advisory Council for the State of Illinois, and an advocate and educator of brain-injury issues for over eighteen years

"The story of Brian's courageous battle to survive and to regain the life he knew before his brain injury is told here eloquently and often with surprising humor. Ever since I have known Brian, it has been his goal to advocate for those who, like himself, are facing the grueling day-to-day challenges of life with a brain injury. With this book he has now become a voice for the millions whose lives have been changed forever, in an instant, by a TBI. Perhaps their best hope is a world that understands. Brian's story takes us a step in that direction, providing a rare, totally honest, and insightful view of what is incomprehensible to most of us."

-Linda Muller, former vice-president, Cognitive Rehabilitation Specialists

every 21
seconds

every 21 seconds

brian d. sweeney

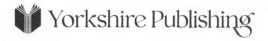
Yorkshire Publishing

ISBN: 978-1-946977-91-5
Every 21 Seconds
Copyright © 2009 by Brian D. Sweeney

Yorkshire Publishing
3207 South Norwood Avenue
Tulsa, Oklahoma 74135
www.YorkshirePublishing.com
918.394.2665

dedication

This book is dedicated to those who understand and is intended for those who do not.

Special thanks to my brother John, who helped edit this book.

foreword

Anything can happen.

Anything can happen, at any time.

Anything can happen, at any time, anywhere.

Anything can happen, at any time, anywhere, to anyone.

While crossing the street, you can be struck by an oncoming car. You can lose your balance while hanging up Christmas lights and fall. The same can happen as you clean the gutters. The forklift at work can overturn and eject you onto the pavement. A high-placed box can fall on you. You can, like many athletes, be injured while playing sports. Or like Brian, you can be the victim of violence.

These are just some of the scenarios that can lead to brain injury and, in less than a New York "second," life can be altered forever. Persons that have suffered a brain injury as well as their families know full well the breadth and scope of the impact on self and family. They know full well the effects on social and work life, the continued drain on the family's finances, and the high rate of divorce. They also know the psychological ups and downs that the injured person can have, the uncontrollable anger, frustration, depression, and anxiety that, like a tsunami, appear and disappear, leaving a void, confusion, and misunderstanding in its wake. They also know that, unlike other diseases, a brain injury is forever with ongoing sequela. Insomnia can present itself almost immediately, making all the other issues worse. Memory issues and personality changes can manifest themselves months after the injury and wreak havoc. In addition, there are numerous physiological and anatomical changes that have filled many medical tomes.

They also know the misunderstanding that can occur in the workplace with friends, relatives, and society as a whole. The mislabeling as malingering or symptom amplifier. Perceptions and notions that are reinforced by cartoon characters that see birds circling after getting hit with a frying pan, movie characters making remarkable recovery in full makeup, or the person who magically awakens but conveniently has selective amnesia of only the bad past events. Reality, in this case, is much more complicated than the movies. Complexities, sequela, barriers, and difficulties are many. From a treatment point of view, brain injury is grossly misunderstood, unrecognized, underdiagnosed, often misdiagnosed or not understood. Therefore, it is commonly mistreated or untreated.

In the following pages, Brian Sweeney gives by far the best personal account and understanding of the realities faced by people with brain injury and their families that I have encountered. He approaches all facets of his injury and recovery with sincerity and visceral strength that is seldom witnessed. What started as a work of soul searching and therapy has become a noble and impressive story of the human spirit in the face of inner turmoil and outer adversity. His struggles, efforts, and experiences are typical of his injury, and as such this work can be considered the voice of many. With incredible insight that can only be gained by experience, he shares with the reader the unknown path of brain injury in a straightforward and honest manner, providing knowledge, understanding, and guidance that is unmatched in scientific textbooks, lectures, or articles.

Readers will also notice the similarities between Brian's story and stroke, as well as Parkinson's and Alzheimer's diseases, autism, multiple sclerosis, cerebral palsy, and brain tumors. The pathology that affects the human brain by far outnumbers any other human disease, and currently there are over 17 million Americans facing issues similar to Brian's. This number is greater than the combined population of New York City, Chicago, Miami, Houston, and Los Angeles. Moreover, this number is expected to increase as our veterans return from the Middle East and the baby boomer population ages. A truer definition of the word epidemic cannot be found.

In reference to traumatic brain injury, the title says it all: *Every 21 Seconds*, signifying the frequency of brain injury in the United States. In the three minutes it will take to read this foreword, approximately nine traumatic brain injuries with all their complications will have occurred, and lives will change. Moreover, this rate will continue on and on. The worldwide numbers are even more staggering: every fifteen seconds.

Unlike a cut of the skin or a broken bone, most brain injuries are not visible. Perhaps, if they were just as obvious as a bruise or laceration, recognition and treatment would be timely, words like malingering would not be used, and insurance companies, employers, and the legal system would be more understanding. In addition, my job as a brain injury doctor would be much easier, and Brian more than likely would not have written these words. Until that time, this book will go a long way in educating those who have not suffered a brain injury and helping those who have.

Of course, the question begs itself: How can a person with a brain injury write such an insightful account? My answer: Read the story.

Ricardo G. Senno, MD, MS, FAAPMR
Diplomate, American Academy of Physical Medicine and
Rehabilitation
Brain Injury Specialist
May 17, 2008

In addition to being an Urban Planner, Dr. Ricardo Senno is a board-certified Physical Medicine and Rehabilitation/ Disability physician with extensive experience in the management and treatment of traumatic brain injury, anoxic brain injury, stroke, movement disorders, and general rehabilitation. His experience includes:

- Having been consulted on numerous medical legal cases, including the Terry Shiavo and Firestone tire cases, he has intimate knowledge of injury-prevention design elements.

- As a recognized expert, he extensively participated in the development of "Heads Up: Concussions in High School Sports" and "Heads Up: Brain Injury in Your Practice" educational kits published by the Center for Disease Control (CDC).

- As Medical Director of the Brain Injury Medicine and Rehabilitation Program at the renowned Rehabilitation Institute of Chicago, he developed seamless patient-care programs and designed a state-of-the-art facility.

- Internationally (Slovenia, Argentina, Sweden, Kuwait) consulted on hospital, clinic, and facility designs.

- Lectured nationally and internationally on facility/space design as it relates to medical management, advocacy, staff utilization, and injury prevention.

- Research and numerous publications dealing with injury prevention, patient evaluation, treatment, recovery, and outcomes following disability.

- Featured in the Chicago Tribune, Sun Times, Daily Herald, Discovery Channel, Telemundo, Univision, and Web MD.

Dr. Senno earned his medical degree from the University of Illinois, completing his internship at Norwalk Hospital (Yale University Medical Center) and his residency at Boston University Medical Center. In addition, he holds a Master of Science in Urban Planning, Public Management, and Policy Analysis. This gives him a unique perspective in the field of Americans with Disability Act (ADA) design and universal architecture and is currently involved in the design and development of the El Valor International Inclusion Center in the Illinois Medical District. In collaboration with colleagues, Dr. Senno is currently writing a book on the issues faced by people with brain injury.

He welcomes e-mails at ricardo@
medicalexpertsandconsultants.com

introduction

When I began writing this story in 1997, I started with a pen and sixty pieces of paper. Eventually, I evolved to a computer, which seemed logical. For some reason, I found this story as amazing as those I told it to did, so it just made sense to write it down. What was amazing to me was that the person I was actually talking about was, for lack of a better term, myself. Far too often I find myself in shock that I have accomplished so much since my injury. There are so many of life's events that we take for granted, all of which once appeared to be out of my reach. As proud as I am about what I have regained, there are times I would like a *do over*. Most of those *do over* moments are episodes that are not happy memories and, unfortunately, came at the expense of those closest to me. However, since the day I started this story, the feeling I experienced while writing was indescribable. I guess I would call it therapeutic.

As the years passed, I continued to add to those sixty pieces of paper. The reason for adding was simple: It seemed that the life experiences I encountered were sometimes altered due to my injury. The injury that happened to me, and to someone in the United States every twenty-one seconds, is a traumatic brain injury (TBI), and the reason I could keep writing is because these types of injuries never go away. I began to believe that a brain injury is the most misunderstood injury one could encounter. How could something that in most cases can't be seen be so devastating? There are parts of your life that fall back into place; however, there are more parts of your life that do not. What is most difficult about living with a brain injury is that your deficits are not on the surface, and you most often feel trapped and, quite honestly, hesitant to voice those deficits or struggles.

Within this book are situations that, quite frankly, would have had completely different outcomes or may have never occurred had I not suffered a traumatic brain injury. However, I did suffer a brain injury, and brain injury survivors too often encounter these types of situations or experiences. The primary reasons these situations occur are twofold. Some of these situations are a direct result of the injury, and others occurred due to a lack of understanding or comprehension of how complicated this injury can be. I was instantly removed from the life I knew and handed a whole new box of challenges. When this injury occurred, I was a married father of two. I had a great career with a great company. I remodeled houses and coached baseball and soccer. I played sports and was in the gym five days a week. I loved my life, and after this happened, I wanted all of it back—not just some of it, but all of it. There was no way you could convince me that I would not be able to do everything I once did. The healing process, if you are fortunate enough to have a healing process, is slow and frustrating. In reality, you never quit healing.

You will read about situations at home and outside of the home that I wish had never happened. I use them as examples of how a brain injury affects one's ability to handle these situations, as well as to identify possible alternatives as to how they could have been avoided. I am sure that if my ability to handle or identify negative situations was not altered, most if not all of the negative effects would not have occurred. Conversely, in certain circumstances a small amount of understanding would have gone a long way.

As the years passed since my injury occurred, I became active in working with others who have suffered a TBI. I offered to meet with brain injury survivors and their families and discuss the "brighter side." I also offered advice based on personal experience. The times where I did have the opportunity to meet with families, the experience was as positive for me as it was for them. There were times when I met the TBI survivor and the family within weeks of the initial injury. To watch family members cry with hope when I would tell them that I suffered a similar injury was quite moving. The feeling I received knowing I was a bright side to a devastating injury was priceless.

I put my family through some very tough times due to my injury. However, we have shared a lot of good years since. I never look back regarding the injury; it happened, so move on and try to enjoy life. My primary purpose for putting this story together was to provide a realistic view into what some of the struggles are for all of us who have endured a brain injury. I also want those who read it to understand that brain injury survivors are still capable of so much; all we require is a bit of understanding and, in some cases, patience. There are 1.5 million traumatic brain injury cases a year; there were 1.5 million last year and 1.5 million the year before that.

I know that no two TBI survivors have the same recovery, and no one ever knows to what degree they will recover. For the most part, I have done quite well, and realizing what I have gone through and having the ability to write about it has helped me tremendously. However, I also know that some of what I have endured has not been very fair, and the bulk of it is due to the fact that the vast majority of the public has no clue what we are going through. Not that they have to; however, I hope what I have written helps, because statistically every twenty-one seconds someone in America suffers a traumatic brain injury. So at any moment, you could join the ranks of the 1.5 million who experience some form of this injury every year. To what extent each one suffers, no one will ever know.

I sometimes feel like I went from a near-perfect life to one I did not recognize. The sad part is, it was harder on those around me than it was on me...initially. The primary reason I wrote *Every 21 Seconds* was to open some minds to exactly what it is we endure. There is so much that is hidden and, in most cases, completely misunderstood. I also wrote it because I felt like there was too much I wanted to say, and this was the only way I could say it. I know others with a TBI who would like me to say this: traumatic brain injuries never go away.

In this book you will see how life changes with a TBI, not just for me, but for those close to me as well. I talk about life experiences and how a TBI impacts those experiences. I talk about everything that I hope makes sense in understanding the effects of a TBI. I discuss work and the impact that negative situations can have on you and your family. The truth is that at times I have let my guard down and believed that what others thought about me may actually be true. There is this hope I have that maybe I can provide some insight into what life really is like with a brain injury. One thing I never wanted was pity; all I tried to do was get back to the life I had and to continue living it. Every time I get the opportunity to meet someone with a TBI, I wonder if they feel the same as me, or if he or she has had some of the same experiences. I wonder if they too have been convinced through negative life situations that they are less than what they once were. From the moment you suffer a TBI, you are in a relearning phase, and you never get to leave that phase. Sure, as time goes on, you recognize progress; however, it has been fifteen years for me, and I still experience deficits, which means I still have to figure out ways to cope with them. You begin to realize what types of life situations you should avoid.

If I am going to enjoy the time I have left, simplicity is a must. As I mentioned, writing this story was quite therapeutic for me. I hope you enjoy reading it and at the same time gain a little understanding about the topic, which has been called the "silent epidemic." It has been called this because traumatic brain injuries are too often not recognized, under-diagnosed, and misdiagnosed. This book is based on a true story—mine. Enjoy the ride.

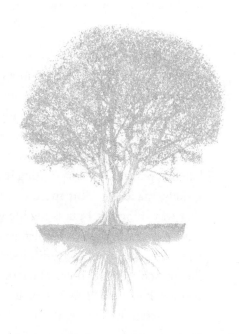

crash and burn

november 2002

I am fairly confident when I say that anyone who began his or her day the way I began this particular November morning would find it completely strange. The sad part is, I did not find anything regarding the following events strange, not this year at least. On this particular day, I woke up around six in the morning with this bizarre collection of paragraphs running through my mind. Based on all that had been going on in my life, I felt compelled to write them down. I ran straight out to my garage, sat in my car, and began writing. As I wrote, the paragraphs that came out were about the life that I was living coming to an end. I knew my life had become one non-stop barrage of bad events, and I was certain that I was going to figure out a way to fix it. However, this batch of paragraphs was pointing in a direction that, quite frankly, made me a bit more confused with everything that was going on. I guess my life was more than a little out of control; it was completely out of control. I just wanted to do something right. Every direction I turned, I dug myself a deeper hole. The strange situations at work had a rollover effect at home, and as home life became more stressful, I brought that stress to work. I really could not win. The poem that I wrote in my car—I guess you would call it a poem—was about watching my own funeral. I believe what I wanted was to somehow stop the pain I felt and the pain I was causing. Although my poem never indicated how I actually passed on, it gave me the opportunity to feel at ease knowing that my life could not get worse. What was odd about this poem—well, actually the whole thing was a bit odd—was that in the poem I was watching over those who came to pay their final respects to me. Of course, there is always the possibility that they were there to stick a pin in me to make sure my batteries had finally run out of energy. The year had been one long string of bad events; actually, *bad* would be an upgrade.

The year 2002 started with me walking out of work just eleven days into January and not returning until sometime in April. Fortunately, or unfortunately, I saw it coming. There seemed to be an arrow pointing at me, at least from one person anyway, and he coincidentally happened to be the person I reported to at my place of employment. This particular company had been my place of employment since 1986. From the first meeting I had with him, there was this strange feeling of *your days are numbered,* and the number is not very high. A week prior to January 11, 2002, I told my wife, Mary Beth, that the tornado was going to strike any day, and I was the trailer park sitting directly in its path of destruction.

I had been hit by a tornado, for lack of better terms, close to ten years earlier and was warned about what I could expect if I was not careful. I was told that as a result of that event, my life and my ability to deal with certain situations like the one I was about to face could be quite hazardous to my health, especially in that region located above the neck and between the ears.

For some odd reason, walking out of my place of employment felt a complete relief. Due to what had occurred ten years earlier, I had to keep notes on what I needed to remember, as well as notes that might prove valuable in circumstances like the one I was facing at work. Anyways, I walked out, got in my car, put on a favorite CD, and drove out of the lot. I was hopeful that I would get a chance in the very near future to tell my side of the story to those who might listen; outside of that I was going to try and figure my life out during this unplanned vacation.

I'll never know why my manager, Ron, or possibly

others as well wanted me out. Was it due to the limitations I had from my brain injury? Or maybe some people just didn't like me; I don't know. I guess it really doesn't matter. The following Monday I was given the opportunity to speak my peace, and I was pretty sure the perception of me this person already had formed was not pretty. This individual's title was Human Relations Manger, and his name was Ted. Ron and I would meet with Ted to review the situation. Ted was close to retirement, very close, so I wasn't so sure this was something he wanted to deal with. During the meeting, Ron stated his reasons for his discontent with me in regards to work, and I provided the documentation I had regarding my experiences at work. My assumption was that under no circumstances would Ted take a side, but he would try to determine a solution to this issue. We both presented our version of the situation, and I left. I really had no desire to stay, and for some reason, I had no planned date for returning. My doctors had recommended that I take a "disability leave."

During the time I was off, my primary physician suggested I talk to someone, someone who gets paid to listen and advise—someone called a psychiatrist. I am sure I met with someone like that years ago following my injury; however, I was a bit apprehensive about meeting with a *shrink*. Maybe I was worried I would find out I had a lot more issues than I had thought. I remember thinking that with all I had going on, this psychiatrist would need a shrink by the time my sessions were complete.

I agreed and met with a female psychiatrist. It actually felt good to open up and talk to someone who wanted to listen. Of course, she was paid to listen, but that is beside the point. This went on for weeks, and I do believe it would have gone on a lot longer if she had had her way. After a few weeks, her recommendation was: "You need to quit where you work before you go insane." Her thought was that I was being mentally beaten. I told her that if I quit, I couldn't pay her bill. She was right; what I was going through at work was wrong, and due to the deficits left over from ten years ago, it was harder to battle. One side effect from having this type of permanent injury was insecurity. It was unbelievable how insecure I had become, and this type of hostile work environment just fueled my insecurity. Every time I had to go into an office to be scrutinized, which seemed to be how the majority of my time was spent, I felt like I was ten years old. I had absolutely no self-confidence; every ounce was gone. Outside of that place I felt fine—well, fine might be an exaggeration, but I will say I felt much better than I did when I was there. I just tried to remind myself that as much as I wanted to run away from this version of the company where I had spent so many years, I had to stay for my kids' sakes. This large company where I had been employed for years suddenly seemed to shrink. The mistreatment I experienced at work was the foundation for the majority of what was going wrong in my life; from there everything else became worse.

Outside of the visits to the psychiatrist, I spent those next three months growing my hair, finishing a few basements, and working out. It just so happens that finishing basements and decks was a sideline of mine.

Those skills were never affected by the injury. I felt quite relaxed, met with some lawyers, and felt good about the meetings, even though I am not a big fan of lawyers. I just wanted to be sure I knew where I stood, and they provided some relief, so I guess I became a fan of those particular lawyers.

During the time I was off, I received a phone call from Ron. The reason he called was to inform me that I was no longer being paid. The fact that I was not being paid didn't bother me; it was the phone call and the tone of his voice as he told me I was no longer being paid that was bothersome. It felt as though he was hoping I would quit. Before I hung up, I asked Ron not to call again, and I told him I would return when my doctors agreed I was ready. The closer the return day came, the more stressed and irrational I became. I somehow got myself together and interviewed with a competitor. At the conclusion of the interview I was offered a position in sales, so I felt good about that part of my life. The interview with a competitor was my way of injecting a feeling of sanity into my life. Truth is, even though this other company seemed to feel I was a good fit based on their limited exposure to me, I knew that if they saw my medical history, they might change their minds. I was always worried about that particular detail. No college degree and being disabled was not a good combo on the job application. However, I was determined not to quit. I had been fighting something that no one could see for ten years, so one more fight couldn't hurt.

While I was out on disability leave, Ted, the

Employee Relations Manager who was involved in this investigation, retired. I really had no reaction to his departure. He seemed somewhat cold to the whole ordeal. His replacement, Earl, had spoken with me by phone and promised to try to resolve this situation to the best of his ability. I will say that as much as I hoped he would be neutral, I was very aware that those to whom I reported would have had all the time they needed to create a visual of who they wanted Earl to believe I was, and what they thought should be done with me. All of those involved worked in the same building and, most likely, had plenty of time to get to know one another. Translation: *I got problems.*

After being out for close to three months, and against my doctor's wishes, I returned to work. This was going to be a reunion neither side was looking forward to. The stress of waiting to see what it would be like was killing me; I just wanted to get what I knew was going to be horrible over. I wished it were the day I left, not the day I was going to return. My drive from home to work was about thirty-five miles; typically, there was heavy traffic and I caught every red light. On the day I returned to work, the traffic was extremely light, almost non-existent. And the red lights? There weren't any. I might be exaggerating here, but it seemed like the commute took about two minutes. On the one day I would have appreciated some red lights and traffic jams, no such luck.

I have to say that the day I returned to work was a test of how much mental torture one can handle. I sat in my car in the parking lot staring at the building. Life had become one huge nightmare, and going in there took every ounce of guts that I had. When I arrived, I had to wait in the lobby, which felt strange. Once inside I met with Tony, my manager's manager. Tony gave me a rather dismal overview of my future with the company. I expected nothing different; a "Welcome Back" banner would have been nice, but this was more in line with what I anticipated. Now I knew Tony was frustrated with this situation and, most likely, wished his time was being spent on something more productive, so I was expecting to hear some comments that might have been the result of his frustration. However, I just kept thinking, *This can't be happening.* You see, I worked in a one-story building, which was referred to as the region office. It was like another world compared to the rest of the company. Anyway, the walk over to my department felt like traveling through a war zone holding a "shoot me" sign. By the time I arrived at the door to my department, I felt about six inches tall. I just wanted to quit, I really did. One thing that kept me from quitting was the picture of my family that I kept in my shirt pocket; those five faces were the reason I could not quit. I loved them more than I hated the situation. The only good thing upon my return was that one of the staff members pulled me into his office and told me that what had gone down appeared to be personal toward me and was, in his opinion, handled horribly. He said that he was there if I needed to talk. The only problem was that as much as I appreciated his comments, I knew that what was ahead of me was not going to be pretty.

Prior to having a *welcome back* meeting with my

manager Ron, I was told to meet with Earl, the Employee Relations Manager. Again, he was new to the position, and I had never met him before. I don't recall anything significant about the meeting outside of two particular directives that Earl gave me. The first was that I was not to have contact with certain individuals within the company, specifically a former manager who had become a good friend. He was a vice president with the company and was now domiciled on the West Coast. I was told that I was no longer allowed to have contact with him; no phone calls made to or accepted from that individual. I just nodded. The second directive from Earl was to *never bring up my disability at my place of employment.* Now, that directive struck me as stranger than the first one; however, again I just nodded in agreement. I don't know why I was told to never mention my disability. The vast majority of those domiciled in the building I worked in never knew I had a traumatic brain injury, nor did I find it necessary to mention the fact that I had a disability. Maybe they wanted to keep that quiet; I just didn't know. Like I said, I didn't fight either directive; I just kept hoping the clock would move faster. If I wasn't so intimidated by returning to work, I do believe I would have questioned what I was told out of curiosity. For all I know, Earl may have been told to bring those two directives to my attention. He did tell me that the walk over to the part of the building where my department was would most likely be the longest and worst walk I had ever taken. Earl was one hundred percent right on that one. That was the bulk of this meeting. Now off to more motivational meetings.

I made it to my department and was then told to meet with the originator of this mess, my manager Ron. I just sat down and tried to prepare myself for what was coming. Ron told me they had replaced the computer equipment I had been using prior to leaving (it appeared I was given the oldest and slowest computer available), and he told me that from that point on I was to write down everything I did and what time that I did it. He wanted me to document everything I did from the minute I arrived at work to the minute I left. He wanted it done every day, and at the end of the day I was to bring the list to him, sort of like a management time card.

Ron also gave me some good news. As was the case every year for management, March was the increase-in-pay month. Now an increase in pay was not the first thing I was wondering about when I returned; as a matter of fact, it was the last item on my list. Anyway, he so eloquently told me that I was being given an increase in my monthly pay, and that increase was twenty-five dollars. Now I do believe that any increase in pay, regardless of size, should always be appreciated, and this certainly was appreciated. However, for some reason he found it absolutely necessary to tell me that it was the lowest amount possible he could give me, followed by: "I didn't even want to give you that." I had to hear, "I didn't even want to give you that," repeated at least five times. The last time Ron said it, he explained why he had even bothered to give me an increase. He told me that in the event I somehow, someway, qualified to receive a management bonus at the end of the year, I had to have been given an increase in pay in order to qualify. I endured his verbal abuse and left. The truth was Ron lost. Not that I won, because I certainly never felt like a winner. It's just that I was still there, so he lost. His mission was to get me out of the company, and he was not successful. The department manager Tony (Ron's manager), who I referred to earlier, was stuck in the middle of this mess. He was new to our region and had walked right into this. In all honesty, he did an excellent job and was most often perceived as fair. I told him that one day he would see a different side of me, not just the skewed version of me described to him by Ron. I didn't hold anything against Tony except that I wish he would have recognized this situation for what it truly was, and he did not. Then again, maybe he did and chose to support Ron, who worked for him, which I can understand. Either way, it doesn't matter. I will say this, in order to avoid just breaking down and throwing in the *employment towel,* I kept trying to imagine that all this was not happening. I had to; otherwise, I would have gone absolutely crazy right on the spot.

I left Ron's office and walked back to my assigned "desk," a corrugated board on top of two filing cabinets, which was located as close to the back door as possible. During the walk back to my desk, nobody said a word to me, not a single word. This went on for weeks. My best guess as to why I received the silent treatment was that the other employees did not want Ron to see them talking to me. This silent treatment felt like something you would experience in grammar school; the only thing missing was recess. Every day was the same for me: I would mark down the hours as they passed, at noon I ran out the back door for my lunch hour, always returning at 12:59, and would bolt out that back door everyday at 5:01 p.m. However, I made sure to give Ron the list of things I had done for the day. The sad part was, I previously had a very successful career there and had proven myself every year, even after my brain injury. I did the best I could after the injury with the strengths that remained. I won multiple awards, was recognized corporately, I made a decent income and then this happens. This whole chain of events was puzzling to me. It felt like Ron had decided that a person with my type of disability no longer belonged, and this was not the first time I felt that way. By the way, one thing I was taught by the therapists was to document everything, which I did, and that helped me win as much of this fight as possible. However, it was nowhere near the end.

After returning to work, the demons between the ears continued to erode my well-being. My behavior was becoming more unusual, and my mood was continually in the mud. Sixteen years at a Fortune-500 company, where I had experienced great success, and now it appeared that my career was coming to an end because I had a TBI. This company had well over a quarter of a million employees at the time and at least two of them did not appear very fond of me, so I figured that two out of 375,000 wasn't bad. As the worst part of returning appeared to be over, I had a feeling that another surprise was lurking just around the corner, and it wasn't going to be a good surprise.

Outside of the normal everyday paranoia my brain was

dealing with at work, something I was not expecting was coming my way. During the time I was out on disability, someone had gone through my desk. I am not sure who or why someone would do this or what he was looking for. What was removed from my desk was a UPS Air Shipping document with my name on it, no credit card number in the billing section, and my work address as the return address. Now the strange thing is, this was among many shipping documents in my desk; and mysteriously this person just happened to choose this one. Shipping personal items this way was a normal procedure for me, and I had done it for years. Every time I had shipped this way, the company sent me a bill and I paid it. This bill was for something personal I had sent right before my three-month sabbatical took place. What was strange was that this particular one had been billed to the company, not to me. Also, this particular shipping document was used for a personal shipment right before I initially walked out, so I never received the bill. The bill would have been shipped to my work address. While I was out, the fact that I made this shipment and never had the bill forwarded to me was the last thing on my mind.

I was called over to Earl's office to discuss this issue. The call came two weeks after I had returned to work. I guess it caught me a bit off guard, but even in the mental state I was in, I found this situation to be somewhat ridiculous. Prior to meeting with Earl, I made a call to the billing department and asked how this one shipping document could have been billed to the company. I had clearly checked "Bill the Shipper," which was me. They had no clue as to how this had happened. I asked them to fax me my shipping history, proving I had no intention other than to receive a bill and pay it. What they faxed over was twelve pages demonstrating that this was exactly the way I had shipped for years, and they had billed me correctly every time.

I met with Earl and provided my billing history. I was sure the information I provided would put this fire out; however, Earl managed to convince me during this meeting that my career appeared over. He said, "It looks like you will not be returning; however, we will do an investigation, and you will be paid during this investigation." I remember telling him, "Doesn't this seem strange to you that the only one incorrectly billed was the one that was taken out of my desk, and all the rest were billed correctly?" He didn't have a reply. At that point I volunteered to take a polygraph test and I offered to pay for it. This request was denied by Earl. With that, I was walked out the door…again.

When I returned home, Mary Beth and I sat in the kitchen, wondering how these individuals could do this. As big as this company was, somebody had to have the brains and integrity to stop this treatment. Two weeks after this fiasco, I was called back to work.

What I am now going to tell you was told to me by a staff member when I returned. What he told me was that my manager Ron had called in a company lawyer to look at the evidence he and Earl had collected against me. The same person who told me that this happened was present at one of the "Sweeney-status meetings," and he said that the lawyer looked at what I had put together versus what was being held against me as evidence and made a very clear statement: "If you are trying to get this company sued, you are doing a great job." Now whether or not that was actually said, I will never know; however, after that meeting, the call came to the house telling me I could return. I was not very nervous coming back this time; the whole chain of events began to seem pathetic, though I always remained confident that one day it would stop; it had to.

I honestly have to tell you that the way these events happened and the way they were tactically carried out would lead me to believe that their intent was to drive me out the door and watch me mentally crumble at the same time. Maybe they just saw me as someone completely different than I saw myself, which is possible. Maybe their opinion was that I didn't belong there any more. The truth was, leaving the company permanently seemed like the only way out of this mess. However, somewhere in my mind, my belief that things would get better was stronger than my belief that they would get worse.

•• •• ••

I was twenty-nine years old when my traumatic brain injury occurred in November, 1992. Since then, I have realized all too well that brain injuries are permanent. There are times when you think you have faced everything a brain injury can throw at you, and then a new set of life's circumstances comes your way, forcing you to face another aspect of a brain injury that you never expected. The type of injury I have inhibits my ability to deal with repeated negative situations. Whether at work or home, it doesn't matter. My mind takes these situations and builds on them. If something negative at work happened, it stayed on my mind constantly, and anything that followed built on it. Maybe the negative occurrences at work were not as bad as they appeared, and my brain injury brought them to another level; I really can't say. Maybe I was the problem, and they didn't have the heart to tell me that I was working somewhere that, based on my injury, I didn't belong. If in fact they saw me as someone with a brain injury who did not fit in their plans, then okay; I could deal with that. I would have preferred and respected just being sat down and told the truth. To put anyone through what I went through was nothing shy of torture and ethically wrong.

The summer came, and things were getting a bit more out of line. The first day of my vacation I tore out all the landscaping around the house, which I had put in five years earlier. Everything was taken out: trees, shrubs, and rocks were removed. I spent four days, non-stop, redoing the landscape; I had no conversations with anyone but obsessed with getting it done and for no real reason. That same week I sold my dream car, a black BMW, also for no reason. I also made sure my will was in order, put money into college funds for my two younger kids, went on an antique shopping spree, and had a few breakdowns. Actually, I think everything I did was due to a breakdown.

As the year progressed, there were more signs that I was close to a mental breakdown. I became a lot more depressed, and my tolerance for stress was down to zero. Waking up, going to work, eating, just living in general felt like a fight. I too often began to wish that I had died ten years earlier; I really did. My kids were walking on eggshells when they were around me. Things I once enjoyed doing had become a challenge. Motivation to exist seemed to be a struggle to find. My kids, no matter what they thought of me at the time, were my motivation. I knew something was wrong and had been warned for years that my resistance to doctor's recommendations and my insistence that I fight this on my own were going to catch up with me. As the situations at work, home, and life in general continued to pose problems, my ability to handle life continued to diminish. When it seemed like my options for life were not rational, I would stare at my youngest son's face, and this was like kryptonite for me. His face coupled with that perfect smile seemed to shed some sunlight on my life. Going to sleep was something I looked forward to, all the time. Once I was asleep, my only hope was that I did not wake up during the night, because going back to sleep was just south of impossible. My racing brain would not let me. When this did happen, I would go downstairs, sit on the couch, and look through the window at the street.

I stumbled through the end of the summer and the fall.

Now it is sometime in November 2002, about six in the morning, and I am in my garage, sitting in my car, writing a poem about watching my own funeral. When you start your day writing about something so strange as your funeral, you wonder what the rest of the day is going to bring. The verses seemed to fly out of my fingers and onto the paper. I know now my subconscious wanted me to do something that maybe somebody would find and realize that I needed someone to talk to, because there was no way I was going to ask for it, not directly.

I wrote this poem, went back in, showered, and was off to work. When I arrived, I typed the poem in Microsoft Word. I figured it looked better in case it was read, and yes, there was someone at work I had planned on giving this to, in the hope that he would let his past take over for me. His name was Victor, a co-worker at my company, and a former Catholic priest whom I trusted. Victor eventually married after leaving the priesthood. Strange how, due to all the clouds surrounding the Catholic Church, leaving to marry a woman makes him look like a hero. Very strategically I placed the poem on the corner of my desk in hopes that he would read it when I called him over. It worked and he read my poem titled "From Above." It went like this:

So this is the new life we all discussed so politely.
From above I watch my family and friends
Listening to the strange comments spoken so lightly
Reminiscing about how I was this, or how I was that,
Ending each comment with, "I know he's happy where he's at."

I guess we all wonder what the end will bring
A dark tunnel, a bright light, or watching heaven's choir sing.

They stare at me as I lie so still
I listen as they whisper, "Doesn't he look at peace,
No longer a member of the life we lease."

There's my kids, I see the tears on their face
I wish I could reassure them
Their dad will be waiting with open arms
When they enter this strange new place.

Next to them are friends, both old and new.
They always claimed I was the first to try life's games
I hope they know I'll see them again,
Though I'll miss them just the same.

I watch them roll me away
Getting me ready for my trip to my final resting place.
Who will I be, who will I see?
I'm not sure if my prayers are still heard.
If they are, I hope my first sight is my dad's smiling Irish face.

My wife of many years wonders where they all went.
She wonders to herself, now that I'm gone, how will her time
be spent.
I hope she can hear me when I say,
Time will put a smile back on her face,
And the kids will fill her empty days.

I hope they know I will miss them all,
And from Above I wish them well.
Was I a good dad, husband, son, brother, friend?
I guess only their time on earth will tell...

"You wrote this?" Victor asked.

"Yes, yes, I wrote that this morning in my car."

"This is excellent," he said.

I remember thinking, *Here it comes, the line I am hoping for. The former priest who studied in Rome with the Pope is going to ask me if I would like to talk. Come on, former Father Victor, show me there is some sign of your profession left inside of you.*

No dice. He placed it back on the desk and walked away. I wanted to ask him if he left the priesthood or if he was kicked out. Victor must have had a lot on his mind, because I know that on any other day he would have recognized the poem as a sign that something was wrong. He was a co-worker I had known for years, and, looking back, I should have asked him to talk. However, there was a little paranoia with most things I was doing at that time. I was back to square one; something had to change. I was scared—just wasn't sure what my mind would think of next.

It was around eleven in the morning the same day, and like an alcoholic who has a moment of clarity, I had one. I called the rehab institute I was assigned to after the accident and asked to speak with Linda Muller. Linda had handled my therapy and kept in contact with me. When she picked up the phone, my words were pretty much to the point.

"I am throwing in the white flag," I said. "I need help." It felt good to finally say those words.

Help was arranged; unfortunately, I would not be able to see the doctor until December 17. The doctor I would see on that December day was a post-brain injury specialist who would hopefully help me understand and get through this part of my life. The problem was that I wasn't going to see him until a week before Christmas—a month away. I was so focused on the appointment that I was marking the days off on a calendar like a kid counting down the days until school is over. A month was a month too long, and I knew that was just enough time for something to go completely wrong. I felt like a ticking time bomb, and I did not want to blow up. I guess somewhere inside of me, I knew the stress of my life coupled with the aftereffects of my brain injury were going to get the best of me.

Thanksgiving fell somewhere between my request to see a doctor and the day I was scheduled to see a doctor. Normally, Thanksgiving was a pretty quiet day around my house, but not this year. It was right around eleven in the morning, and the time I feared had arrived. In a fit of desperation I called my brother-in-law, Jon Popp, who lived four doors away.

"Jon," I said quietly into the phone, yet with a bit of desperation, "you have to get down here. You have to get down here!"

"What happened? Is everything okay?" Jon replied.

"Just get down here. Something is wrong," I quietly screamed.

Jon left his house and ran up to my door just as the police arrived.

As the officer exited his car, Jon asked, "What's going on?" The officer looked at Jon and replied, "No idea.

Probably nothing." This being Thanksgiving, and Jon having no other thought than maybe someone slicing the Thanksgiving turkey had cut their finger, he grabbed a bottle of wine before he ran down to the house. No Band-aids; just wine. I will admit that there is a bit of humor here—my brother-in-law running down the street alongside the police car with a bottle of wine is a bit comical—but it didn't seem like it then. As Jon and the police officers reached the front door, the ambulance could be heard approaching the house.

As the police entered, they encountered a family of all ages in a bit of shock. There was Jim, sixteen, sitting on the couch with his mop-top in a bit of disarray, and his mom, Mary Beth, holding him while she repeatedly asked, "Are you okay?" Behind Jim's mom was his sister Katie, seventeen, comforting the youngest two, Brian, seven, and Jennifer, five.

"What happened here, miss?" asked the officer.

Mary Beth looked at Jim, hesitated, then replied, "He fell—he just fell...in the hallway."

"Is that what happened, son?" asked the officer.

"Yeah," said Jim. "I...I fell. I got knocked out when I fell. I feel better now." Looking at Jon, the officer asked, "You the dad?"

"No, no, I'm the uncle. I live a few doors down."

"Where is the father?" the officer asked.

Mary Beth said, "He is upstairs." As the paramedics began to look at Jim, Jon shot upstairs in search of yours truly.

"What happened?" Jon asked as he came into the bedroom.

"I knocked him out when we hit the floor," I said through tears. "As both of us went down, Jim hit his head on the floor. I didn't hit him. I just snapped," I replied. "I suppose they will take me in for this."

Jon was staring at me somewhat puzzled; then he asked, "Did you see your head?"

"What are you talking about?" I replied.

"Your head. Look in the mirror. There is blood all over the side," Jon said.

"That is all I need," I mumbled. "I must have slammed it on the coffee table when I fell. Do the police know I am up here?"

"Yeah," Jon replied, "and you should stay until they leave."

I tried to stay as calm as possible while explaining the mess.

"Jon," I said, "I have no idea what is going on with me. This whole year has been bizarre. I am sinking. Work is a prison. It's killing me; has been for a few years. Kids think I'm nuts. Wife is way confused. I am in a state of mind I can't get out of. I called the rehab center last week. You know, the one where I was after the accident, and told them I am throwing up the flag. I will do whatever it takes. I know I am dying inside, and I can't stand it. I've got an appointment with that brain injury doctor in December; it's just not soon enough. I've known that something is wrong for a while. No appetite, up all night, weird thoughts. Now look what I've done. This isn't me, and it hasn't been me since that injury!"

"Hold this rag to your head while I go downstairs," Jon said.

I stood around the corner at the top of the stairs, listening to the paramedics talk to Mary Beth.

"He seems fine. Just keep and eye on him."

Thank God they didn't ask for me to come down.

The morning had started off quite normal, I guess. It was Thanksgiving. Company was to arrive later in the day, and things seemed a bit hectic but fine for the most part. The last few months had been hard on me, and I am sure a bit hard on the family as well. Actually, the year in general had been a complete disaster. The morning was okay until I opened my mouth, and in the angry tone, which Mary Beth had become accustomed to, I impolitely asked, "Do Katie and Jimmy do anything around here?"

Looking at me with the standard head tilt, she replied, "They are fine. Would you just relax?"

Not long after that, Mary Beth's mom called, and as I walked into the kitchen, I heard her begin to tell her mom, "Those older two do nothing around here."

As she continued, the blood began to boil. Just then Jimmy walked up the stairs, and I let him hear it. "You better start helping out around here, Jim, or I am taking the car away." *Taking the car away* was my standard threat, and it never worked because the kids knew I wouldn't do it. Mary Beth hung up quite quickly.

"What is your problem?" she asked.

As the rage began to creep into its middle stage, I

screamed, "I am sick of it! They do nothing and get everything!"

(Quick side note: When depression, courtesy of a brain injury, has its grips on you, nothing makes you happy, and everything in your own domain makes you angry.)

As Mary Beth spoke, Jimmy stared at me. I walked up to him. We were face-to-face; he stood about an inch or two taller, and I just lost it. Mary Beth knew a snap was coming, and boy, did it. As I lunged toward him, she tried to get between us in an effort to slow me down. I grabbed hold of Jim and he grabbed hold of me, and the three of us went down. *Slam!* went my head right on the coffee table. I could hear the bells screeching through my head, and the rest was a blur. Mary Beth said I got up with such rage that it frightened her. I grabbed Jim with uncontrollable anger, picked him up, and threw him to the ground. I can remember the little ones crying and screaming, "Stop, Dad, stop!"

As we hit the ground, he was facedown and I was on top of him. As the whole family was hitting and pulling me, I rolled him over—nothing. He was out cold. We all stopped. No screaming, no hitting, nothing. Jim was out cold.

Oh God! screamed my brain. I began shaking him and screaming, *"Wake up!"*

Brian and Jennifer were still crying and swinging away, God love those two. Jim woke up; he was only out for about twenty seconds or less—just enough time for his mom to dial 911. Where was a busy signal at the Mokena Police Department when you needed one? I got up and walked upstairs. You have no idea how confusing this was—all I kept thinking is, *What has happened to me?* I knew the answer to that question.

After Jon left, I headed downstairs quite slowly. I could still hear the kids screaming and crying in my head, though it all ended as I entered the kitchen. The whole family was still in the front room. I made my way to the kitchen and stared out the window. I could feel the tears on my face, but for the most part the only thing I felt, or rather heard, was this voice in my head asking me, *How did this happen?*

I knew the answer and was three weeks away, when I would return to the same hospital I was in ten years earlier to meet with a doctor who specialized in brain injuries. I was hoping, praying that he could help me get my life back on track. I sat there thinking how ironic it was that exactly ten years ago this very week my life was derailed. I relive that event one way or another every day of my life. It is amazing that something no one can see is so devastating. Traumatic brain injuries occur every twenty-one seconds, and like they say, you never see it coming. I absolutely agree with that statement. Let me take you a back a few years.

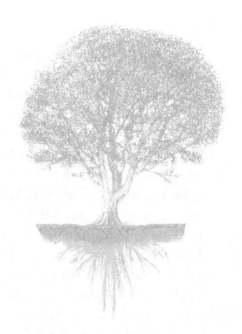

life as i knew it

november 1992, chicago, illinois

Up until the time I was in my late teens, I thought any place other than the south side of Chicago was nothing more than a place to visit. For the most part, I had a fairly simple childhood. I was the fourth of five children, we grew up on a city street filled with kids, and we all attended the same Catholic grammar school, St. Christina.

I lucked out and was given a Schwinn Continental bicycle for my Confirmation. Most kids got the Schwinn

Varsity, but I think I drove my dad crazy just being around him, so he figured the nicer the bike, the farther away I'd go. I have to admit, it was a clever plan. I guess I was different than my brothers; as a matter of fact, I know I was different. My brothers and my only sister thought there were two things in life: school and baseball, and school came second. Me, I wasn't into baseball, at least not as much as most kids. Sure, I played, but with no real commitment. I was more into tearing things apart and putting them back together or rebuilding old bikes that I found in the trash. As I got older, I was the one you called to install a cassette player in your car, or if your car needed brakes, I was the guy. On a few occasions I was asked to break into my neighbors' houses when they had locked themselves out. I'm not sure why they would ask me to do that; maybe they thought I had locksmithing in my future. Or maybe they thought I would be a...no, I'm sure they were thinking locksmith or window cutter.

As I got older, I discovered a new joy: planning trips, or as they are sometimes referred to, *road trips*. Whether it was a trip to Schaffer Lake, Indiana, with the boys or renting local hotel suites under false names, you could count on me. Somehow, I always seemed to be the one who went a bit overboard to make sure everyone had a great time; not that I didn't, it's just that for some odd reason it was more important to me that others have a better time. Some would call that being a "people pleaser"; I just figured I was good at making sure others were entertained.

I seemed to get bored easily. Coming up with things

to do that were a bit unusual seemed to get the adrenalin cooking. Bob, a friend I had through my teens and early twenties, used to say, "You are always the first." I was the first one to get a car, and the first one to sell a car. I was the first one to get a checking account, and the first thing I bought, and Bob was with me, was the classic electric football game that would vibrate the players down the field. Nice first purchase, and believe it or not, twenty-something years later I still have that game. I was the first one to move out, and the first one to move back.

I called Bob one day and asked him to meet me at Big Mickey's hamburger joint so I could spring another *first* on him. I had to tell someone, and at the time he was my closest friend. I looked him straight in the eye and said, "Bob, get ready for this one....I'm getting married." Coincidentally, it was to a girl I had met at one of the *hotel parties* I had thrown a couple years back. If I had to write a list consisting of the best firsts, this one would take the cake.

The *firsts* continued: first to have one kid, first to have two, the first to get a house, and so on. No matter how many of life's events I encountered, when I least expected it, the *worst first* came, and at a time when I thought those days were over.

The only thing typical about this November, 1992 weekend was the weather. The boys and I had been planning this road trip for weeks. This was our Bi-Annual Boys Only weekend at my in-laws' cottage in Lake Geneva, Wisconsin. Lake Geneva was Wisconsin's version of Las Vegas, minus the gambling. My partners on the trip were four friends I had known most of my life. We all grew up together in a small part of Chicago's southwest side. It was an Irish Catholic, blue-collar, sports-loving, beer-drinking neighborhood known as the infamous Mount Greenwood area. It seemed like the majority of the neighborhood was comprised of City of Chicago employees. My dad was one of those city employees; he was one of Chicago's finest, a Chicago police officer. Most of my neighbors, as well as my friends' fathers, were either Chicago police officers or Chicago firemen. Mount Greenwood was the type of neighborhood where you knew everyone, and you were asked to abide by the Mount Greenwood laws. Those laws state that since you were born and raised in Mount Greenwood, you must stay there. You preferably marry someone from the neighborhood, and she should be a friend with one of your friends' future wives. That makes the whole "hanging out with the same guys you grew up with" a lot easier. The two of you would raise your kids there, keep the same friends (forever), and for God's sake, don't ever move. It was and still is a great neighborhood. Personally, I only paid attention to the first two, the *born and raised* laws. By the way, if you do move, which is frowned upon, sell your house to a fireman or policeman.

One of the local Mt. Greenwood customs that I always found somewhat funny was the way by which you would typically have been judged or described when your name was mentioned in conversation. Here is how it worked: Grades, looks, manners, brains, or anything else one would ordinarily find to be personally appealing were never to be considered as primary reasons to judge someone positively or negatively. There was just one measure: baseball, or for that matter any sport, but in Mount Greenwood it was mostly baseball. If you, post-baseball, became a Nobel Peace prizewinner, lived a life of crime, saved a life, had a perfect grade-point average, became the president of the United States, or cured cancer, it wouldn't matter. How well you hit during your Mount Greenwood baseball career was the barometer for life. You would always be defined by sports, specifically your Greater Mount Greenwood Baseball League batting average. My dad was always the gauge for knowing how I did; if I made an out and he gave me a one-hand brush away, it was a good hit; they just caught it. If I got the two-hand brush, I was walking home. Eventually, I just took my bike, the Schwinn Continental, to my baseball games. One more thing about Mount Greenwood: if you grew up there, you will always have a special attachment to the neighborhood and to others who grew up there. And hey, you can always exaggerate your batting average.

Although we were somewhat older now, we viewed these trips no differently than we had twenty years before; of course, we used bikes then, and we had to be home by a certain time. But for the most part, it was the same guys I would have been with at ten years old. It's funny, but as our car inched its way toward good old Wisconsin, the conversation slowly moved from modern day to our childhood. We started out talking about marriage, jobs, kids, and by the time we passed the "Welcome to Wisconsin" sign, we were fighting over musical selections and reliving some of the most unusual stunts pulled by ourselves or friends on past road trips. Of course, if it was a stunt that you were responsible for, it always had to be told by someone else. That way you were made to feel even more moronic than when the actual stunt occurred. These trips typically lasted no more than three days, but during those three days, we were always laughing. Work didn't matter, age was irrelevant, and we just seemed to disconnect ourselves from the pressures of no longer being a kid. I loved those trips.

The most senior member of the group was Kevin Ashe at thirty-three. If they cloned Norm from "Cheers," Kevin would be the result. Nicknamed "Emit," Kevin was single, owned his own company, as well as a tavern and several other endeavors. He has a heart of gold, is a genuinely nice person, and does not have a violent bone in his body. Outside of the fact that he hopes shag carpeting makes a comeback so he doesn't have to remodel his house, he treats himself and those he calls his friends pretty well. Kevin has friends from the age of twenty-five to eighty-five. Quick story about how thirsty Kevin can get. We were golfing once and Kevin decided to sit out the back nine. When we came into the bar to get him, he turned to the bartender and asked for his bar bill. The bartender replied, "Two dollars a beer…forty-eight dollars, please." Kevin looked at us and mumbled sarcastically, flashing his patented grin, "I got issues."

Next on the list was Henry McPhillips, twenty-nine years of age and married. He was a stockbroker for many years and was always up for a good time. He had definitely been looking forward to getting away since he hadn't been on this trip in ten years. I hadn't seen much of Henry in recent years, so I will admit that I was somewhat surprised he was going. Also along for the trip was Henry's younger brother, Tim. Tim was twenty-seven, and we referred to him as "TP." Tim, like Henry, was tall and lanky, extremely polite, and absolutely hysterical when the mood was right. Tim was newly married, an electrician, knew every tune from the fifties, and still believes that Elvis is alive. Tim seemed to come alive if there was a theme behind an event. No matter what the event, the number one question from all attending was, "Will TP be there?" Tim used to drag this mannequin around, actually half a mannequin. Tim named him Eugene. He took him to restaurants, weddings—you name it. By the way, Eugene, for lack of a better term, stood up in Tim's wedding. This alone should make you wish you were with us, or maybe it makes you glad you weren't.

Joe McAvoy, twenty-eight, was also a newlywed and an electrician like Tim. When you thought of Joe, the first thing that came to mind was his loyalty, especially to the Cubbies. To me, Joe, who was always a good time, was the perfect final touch to this boys' trip. Joe always stuck with the basics when it came to wardrobes or cars. Joe liked his cars made in America and his wardrobe simple, as long as it was comfortable. Joe always went along with the program, as long as the program included having fun, and he had a knack for keeping things simple. Plus, he had just been married two months earlier, so he said he needed a short vacation.

As I mentioned earlier, I was always the one throwing the party or planning the trip. I was never good at sitting still. Kevin's dad always said that any bizarre event had me behind it. At that time I had two young children, Katie and Jimmy.

I also like to keep everything I own in its original condition. Whether it is a car, a lawnmower, or a house, it doesn't matter; I have to keep everything I own in perfect condition. I still have that Schwinn Continental I received when I was twelve, and yes, it is in perfect condition. I had been married to Mary Beth since I was twenty-one. Mary Beth was always the logical one. I was the dreamer and still am. I just figured the more dreams I had, the better my chances of one actually being realized. Mary Beth always thought things through. She was so pretty and still is. If I had a dime for every time I heard "How'd you get her?" I could have retired years ago. Mary Beth was the middle one of three sisters. She was very independent and relied on no one. Ever since the day I met her she was independent minded and somewhat on her own.

I have been employed at United Parcel Service (UPS) since I was twenty-three. How I ended up working at UPS was pure luck. I had been driving a truck for a marble company and was barely making ends meet. At the time I had a one-year-old baby and another on the way, and we were broke. We were somehow able to get enough money for a down-payment on a house we bought from my brother Mike. We put every dime we had down on the place, and at the time I was making seven dollars, thirty-five cents an hour, so there weren't a lot of dimes to put down. My brother Steve had applied to work as a UPS package car driver. When they called to offer him the job, he declined because he had recently been offered a job as a police officer and was preparing to enter the police academy. After telling this to my brother Mike, Mike recommended that he call them back and ask if I could have the interview. When I walked in the door, Mary Beth said, "UPS called to see if you would be interested in driving a truck." I thought to myself, *UPS, UPS...oh, the brown trucks.* Sure I would, so I called and scheduled my interview for the following day. All went well, and I was hired as a driver.

After almost a year, they asked me to interview for a management position in sales. I had nothing to lose, and the job appeared to be a good fit. Low and behold, I was awarded the position of account executive. Of course, this meant I had to buy and wear a suit—suits are something I am not a big fan of. However, the opportunity was great. UPS was good to me from day one.

This particular weekend getaway with the friends began with me dropping the kids off at my parents' house while Mary Beth was working. Upon leaving my parents' house, my mom pleaded with me to stay home. On my way out of my mom's house all I heard was, "I got a bad feeling about this, Brian. All you guys do on these trips is drink beer. Why don't you just stay home with your wife and kids?" I laughed on the way out the door. She said that exact same thing every time; however, this time she went a bit overboard, listing all the reasons we should not go. I'm not sure I ever gave her a reason not to worry; she was pretty much right on most accounts.

We all met at Kevin's house and piled into his white 1989 Lincoln Town Car. I volunteered to drive. Coincidentally, I was remodeling Kevin's house at the time. I was converting what was a garage into a family room and was on the last step, the most important step: building the bar. Kevin suggested that we stop at 7-Eleven before we headed north. I had a bad feeling about this first stop. The four ran in and returned with a cheap cooler, ice, and a case of twelve-ounce alcoholic beverages commonly referred to as beer. I popped the trunk from the inside, assuming they would put what they bought in the trunk. The four of them walked right past the open trunk. I kind of laughed, got out, shut the trunk, and asked Kevin if grabbing a case of beer was a good idea. He had his usual sarcastic response, "You're right. One case might not do it. Hey, Joe, run in and grab another case." I just shook it off and said, "You guys do your thing and I'll refrain and drive." One of them mumbled that that would leave more for them.

The trip to Wisconsin was always interesting. Every ten miles we seemed to become a bit less attached to all our responsibilities. We forgot about work, bills, what my mom said, and just seemed to lose a few years, and it was mandatory that the same music we listened to when we were eighteen was on hand for the trip.

We stopped for lunch outside of Lake Geneva at place called the "Brat Stop." This place was a taste of what the real Wisconsin was all about. Packers' signs were everywhere, and every type of cheese made was sold there. We stayed for about an hour and then proceeded to the cottage.

When we arrived, I called every cab and limo company in Lake Geneva. However, each company only had one vehicle, and there were none available. I volunteered to be the designated driver, which meant I would drink half of what the rest did. Typically, that plan worked for about the first half-hour. So off we went to the dog track. While at the Geneva Dog Track, we lost some money, had a few beers, and, as always, verbally abused each other. We left the track at eleven that evening and headed to a bar down the street from the cottage called "Reilly's North." I had been in there several times over the years. This place was a Wisconsin postcard. It was a small dump nestled in the woods and generally was not crowded. The jukebox hadn't been updated since Jimmy Carter was in office. That night though, they had a karaoke, so it was busy. God forbid you missed the opportunity to sing "Paradise by the Dashboard Light," which, fifteen years after it came out, was still listed under the "new releases" column.

We arrived there about 11:15 and were greeted with a *you're not a local* stare by what looked like a sea of John Deere hats. No big deal. We proceeded directly towards the bar. As drinks were ordered, I requested "Cotton Fields," an old Creedence Clearwater Revival tune, for our karaoke song. Ten minutes later we were called. Henry, Tim, Joe, and I went up, while Kevin stayed seated at the bar. We did our thing, two on each microphone.

We stirred up a few laughs and a few stares. Afterward, Henry and Kevin ventured to the men's room.

While we listened to the next person onstage, a fight started at the entrance to the men's room. I noticed that Henry was a part of it and was being pushed out the door, while Kevin was trying to be a mediator. Henry's not a fighter and didn't even know what caused the problem. Joe and I immediately went over and told him to get back to the bar, which he did. We sat down, but we could see that the trouble was not going to stop. Even though we had nothing to do with it, we decided to finish our drinks and head out of there.

As it turns out, the individual causing the commotion was a local man, Nick Smith. My wife vaguely knew him from her childhood days spent at the cottage. He was at the bar with his wife and her friend. Smith was asked to leave by the bar employees for being unruly. After throwing his drink at the female bartender, he agreed to leave. Smith was tall, skinny, and had long black hair and a beard. The bartender and bouncers escorted him outside. However, he headed back in to get his wife *(I guess he forgot about her)*. The bartender greeted him at the door with profanities, and Smith greeted her with his fist. He knocked her out cold. After seeing this, the other employees and some patrons brought Smith outside the bar for an attitude adjustment. It was at this point that my friends and I decided to leave. The last thing I remember was putting on my jacket and heading for the door.

I was told that as we walked out there was a small brawl off to the right of us, but we kept walking towards the car. I trailed behind my friends. Nick Smith emerged from the brawl somewhat enraged and incoherent. The locals and a few employees had given him a good beating. We happened to be walking to the car as the fight ended, and I was the last of the five of us. Smith assumed that we were part of the group pounding on him and made his way towards us. He ran up behind me and struck me with an upward jolt to the back of my head. I dropped like a rock. I assume that I never saw or heard him coming. Smith proceeded to jump on Henry, screaming, "I am going to break your neck!" The other three removed Smith from Henry as the police arrived on the scene. Someone had called the police prior to the bar employees dragging Smith outside. A female bar patron stood over me so the police would not run me over on the side of the street—I appreciated that. One of the bar patrons and the lady who had been standing over me tried to wake me as the police attempted to sort out what had happened. Their efforts to wake me were in vain, so the lady approached Kevin and asked him if he was with me.

Kevin was shocked to see me lying unconscious on the road—they had not seen me get hit. They also tried to wake me but with no luck. With me still unconscious, Kevin and Joe decided to put me in the Lincoln. They each grabbed an arm, dragged me across the gravel road, and laid me in the back seat. An Officer Garner walked over and asked how I ended up on the ground. The lady who had been standing over me when the police turned the corner was the sister of the female bartender whom Smith had knocked out, and she had run outside in pursuit of him in an effort to obtain his license plate number. "That guy hit him!" she said, pointing at Smith. With that being said, the police placed Smith in custody for questioning.

While the boys were being questioned, Officer Garner asked if I was a diabetic, due to my rather loud snoring. He had witnessed that kind of snoring with people in a diabetic coma. Kevin replied that I wasn't. While Officer Garner continued to talk to Kevin, Joe very skillfully removed the twenty-four empty beer cans from the backseat floor. Just as he finished tossing the last one into the bushes, another officer approached Joe and pointed toward the empties. "Yours?" he asked. Joe looked over at the pile and responded, "Those, oh, no, those aren't mine."

The officer had called an ambulance. I have to tell you that this bar, Reilly's North, was a classic. It was in the middle of all these cottages, just sitting there on a dirt road. Absolutely a local bar, it had been there for years with one light in front of it; you know, that ugly fluorescent light that stands about fifteen feet in the air and casts a strange light in only one direction. It was the kind of place where beer in bottles was an upgrade.

Joe McAvoy accompanied me in the ambulance while the other three went back into the bar and had a few cold beers with the employees and patrons who were involved in the "mixed-up-no-martial-art-skills brawl." They stayed there until the police took them back to the cottage. From what I was told, the drive back to the cottage was quite humorous. The house we were staying at was difficult to find if you were not familiar with it, and the remaining three knuckleheads spent an hour in the back of a squad car, with the officer threatening to either drop them off where they were or bring them to the station if he didn't find the damn house. Keep in mind that the cottage was only three blocks from the bar. No charges were filed against Nick Smith that night, and the police escorted him home. The policeman, it turns out, was a childhood friend of Smith's.

I arrived at a trauma center in Elkhorn, Wisconsin, at ten minutes after one in the morning. As they wheeled me in, Joe said the doctor commented, "Another drunken casualty from the Geneva strip." Joe disputed that remark, arguing that there had been a fight at the bar and I was struck in the head while walking to the car. Knowing Joe, he most likely worded that last statement a bit differently, but I'm sure you get the picture. Because I had been at a bar, the doctor assumed I was intoxicated. I suppose he also assumed that I normally bled from the back my head. No testing was performed. I was given an IV and placed in a room to sleep it off.

My wife, Mary Beth, was not notified until Sunday morning. When she was contacted, the nurse had told her, "We believe that Brian is sleeping off a hangover, so you can pick him up later. He should be released by noon."

Mary Beth replied that although I like to have a couple of beers once in a while, it would be out of character for me to drink enough to pass out, let alone not move for what had been about ten hours. The nurse said that the hospital was considering doing a cat scan, since I was incoherent and could not walk. Sounds like this hospital had a pretty sharp staff; imagine having the ability to call for a cat scan when all you have to go on is a head that was bleeding hours earlier coupled with the inability to walk or stay awake. I lucked out. My wife called the cottage and spoke to Kevin, who told her that he had called the hospital and they told him that I was okay and that she would be picking me up.

My wife notified my family of what had happened and was preparing to get me. My brother Steve, a police officer, was skeptical and wanted to make sure everything was okay, so he called the hospital to talk to me. Steve didn't mind mixing it up when he was younger, and had a true belief in the "don't do the crime if you can't do the time" theory. He was an absolute pain in my side while we were growing up; however, Steve always looked out for me. The nurse told him that I couldn't get up because I was drowsy and there was no phone in my room, but I was doing well. The nurse also informed Steve that she was able to wake me up and I had told her that I worked at Citibank and had two daughters. Steve was not happy, because that information was absolutely incorrect. I didn't have two daughters and did not work at Citibank. I'm sure Steve politely explained that to the staff.

Steve called Mary Beth and repeated his phone conversation with the nurse. She then called the hospital screaming. They told her they were doing a cat scan and would be finished by the time she arrived in Wisconsin. Before Mary Beth headed north, she had picked up my mother and her father, James. I wonder how many times my mom said, "I told him not to go....I'm sure he'll be fine...damn kid." They arrived at the cottage at one in the afternoon to grab my belongings. When Mary Beth called the hospital to inquire about my status, the nurse asked, "How quickly can you get here?" When Mary Beth asked why, the nurse informed her that I had sustained a subdural brain hemorrhage and that they were preparing me for a transfer to a hospital in Milwaukee via helicopter (weather permitting, since a snow and ice storm was occurring at the time). They were unable to treat me due to the severity of my condition.

I was transferred via an Intensive Care Transfer Unit to a trauma center in Milwaukee and arrived around five that evening. Additional MRIs, cat scans, and tests were administered. I was diagnosed with a subdural brain hemorrhage. The dura (the sack around the brain) was leaking, and the brain was swelling due to the velocity of the initial strike and the impact of the pavement. My brain had sustained lacerations across the front, and the left side and was bleeding. Due to the severity, the initial intent was to have a helicopter move me to Milwaukee; however, the weather would not permit such a move, so an Intensive Care Ambulance was called. My wife and my mom followed the ambulance to the hospital.

Upon entering the intensive care unit, Mary Beth was greeted with this gracious question, "Would you like to complete the organ donor form?" Not "Are you thirsty after your drive? Do you need to use the bathroom?" or maybe something like, "Would you like to know where the phone is located?" No, none of that; they had Nurse Pessimist greet the wife and mom.

The neurosurgeon told Mary Beth that it would be a few days before they even knew if I would make it because the swelling had not peeked yet. He had seen patients with less damage than I had die. And if I did survive, they had no way of knowing to what degree I would recover. The neuro-intensive care unit was where I would call home until a move could be made to transfer me closer to home.

Most of this time I was unresponsive, sometimes being stirred by a deep sternum rub, where someone digs their knuckles into your sternum to stimulate a reaction. I was tied to the bed because I would become combative, as is the case with most traumatic brain injuries. There was swelling to the cranium, which makes you look like a basketball on a toothpick. Due to the fractured skull, bleeding had turned parts of my face purple. This is a very strange stage of the injury; you may say something after being given sternum rubs, your eyes may never open, subconsciously you may occasionally blurt out a statement, and some of these often came out of nowhere, with little to no real meaning. In some cases my comments were inappropriate. For example, there was the time I gave the nurse my personal comments on her breast size as she was leaning over me. Of course, my oldest brother, Mike, thought these were signs I would be just fine. They said my lack of inhibitions were normal for someone who had suffered a brain trauma. I guess if you were going to get Tourette's syndrome, this was as good a time as any. There were times the brief statements were a bit emotional, and that was due to the location of my injury. For whatever reason, I wish I could go back and just watch how I reacted when I was awake. It is quite strange to know that this and hundreds of other situations occurred involving me and I have no recollection of any of them.

I was given a Glasgow coma rating sometime during my arrival at the trauma center in Milwaukee. The Glasgow rating system is designed to determine the depth of a coma. My initial ranking was a six, and that was after eighteen hours. To give you an idea of what that score means, fifty percent of those with a score of less than eight die within six hours.

When I was awakened, though it was always brief, I was only aware of who I was and of the people I recognized, not the time, the place, or what had happened to me. I always wanted to be untied from the bed and to go home. One night I escaped from the intensive care unit while tied to the bed. I pulled out my IVs and catheter and proceeded completely naked out the electric-censored door and down the hallway to a bathroom. I must have dragged my right side, because there was partial paralysis on that side. So naked and dragging the right side, I was not a pretty sight. The nurses followed the trail of blood and found me lying face down on the bathroom floor. I guess, even though I have no memory of ever being in that hospital, I was and still am proud to be the first patient to escape from the intensive care unit. Unfortunately, because of increased swelling, my condition did not get any better.

My family spent Thanksgiving Day in the hospital cafeteria consuming *mystery meat*. My brothers Mike and Steve, my younger sister Marilyn, as well as my dad and last brother, John, were present. John is the brother I have the most in common with. When John had spoken with my mom via phone two days after this happened, she told him, like most disillusioned mothers, that I would be fine. John asked to speak with Mike, and because my father was recovering from a stroke he had suffered months earlier, and Mom is, well, Mom, the doctors had spoken to Mike upon his request. Mike told John, "You best get here quick. The doctors told me they don't see him living past Thanksgiving, and if he pulls through, he will most likely be a vegetable. My mom had told me that she was in the room when Mike had asked the doctor about my prognosis. When the doctor mentioned that I would have limited cognitive function and may be confined to a wheelchair, Mom could not handle it and walked out. The best part was her rationale for walking out: "How could he say you would be confined to a wheelchair, you just escaped from intensive care a few days earlier, so your legs were fine!" Right on, Mom.

My favorite "arriving in the room and seeing me hooked up to every life support system" story was the one about my brother Steve. I was told he walked in, looked at me, took a pair of rubber gloves from the table, ripped them in half, cried a bit, and told Marilyn's husband, Jim, "Get the car."

Kevin had driven up from Chicago and also spent that day with my family. Kevin was considered the mayor of the area we grew up in; if you wanted to know what was going on, ask Kevin. Prior to leaving with Jim to revisit the scene of the crime, Steve told Kevin, "Tell me what happened." Kevin had been Steve's best friend since childhood. Kevin said, "We didn't do a thing to the guy. Brian just happened to be the first one he came across. I never even saw it happen. One minute we're leaving, and the next Brian is sprawled out on the street." The explanation from Kevin just made Steve angrier.

As for my typical demeanor, I'm told that if the nurses were able to wake me, one eye would open, and normally whoever was there with me would hear the same thing from me. I would ask them to hold my hand, and I would only call them by their complete first name—no nicknames, no cutting it short; I would tell them how much I loved them and ask them to rub my head because it was on fire. I am told this would turn on the human tear machine.

I should mention that the other four who accompanied me on this trip went through extreme guilt over what had happened. According to their wives, they would not answer the phone, afraid of what they might hear, and Henry took my situation especially hard. Henry cried for days. He knew that the person who hit me recognized him prior to hitting me, and that I was just a speed bump before he got to Henry. That little bathroom scene was obviously a bit more intense than we thought, though I believe Henry was just in the wrong place at the wrong time. I have always felt bad about how much this affected those guys. It wasn't their fault. To this day they still prefer not to talk about it, and if they do, you can still see it bothers them. I believe they always had the feeling that they could have done something.

The sad thing is, I never see them anymore; brain injuries tend to leave those close to you thinking differently of you, unable to understand the changes. Here is a strange twist: Henry and Tim went to morning mass every day to pray for me, and the name of the priest was Father Sweeney, the same last name as mine.

I have to explain the trip back to Lake Geneva that my brother Steve and brother-in-law Jim took. Jim had told me that from the hospital to the bar where the incident happened, Steve held his loaded gun in his hand. Jim said that the circumstances they were possibly going to encounter were racing through his head; however, the momentum of the situation carried them right to the bar. Steve and Jim arrived at "Reilly's North" around three in the afternoon. Before getting out of the car, Steve asked Jim, "You with me?" to which Jim replied, "Yeah, I'm with you."

As they walked in, Jim said you could just feel the anger and energy go in the door with them. There were several people scattered around the bar, and the two sat down. They ordered something to drink, and a few moments later Steve walked up to every person in the place and asked, "What happened here last Saturday?" Steve was not very quiet with his delivery of that particular question, and as he addressed one person, everyone in the place heard the question. The joint went silent. Jim told me you could hear dust fall. Jim was watching the faces of everyone in there, all the time knowing that if someone got one bit defensive with Steve's questioning, the worst was possible.

Steve finally encountered the owner of the establishment and without hesitation asked him, "What happened here last Saturday?" Jim said he was sweating, absolutely convinced that something bad was going to happen. With a bit of arrogance, the bar owner said, "From what I understand, these guys from Chicago came up here, and it sounds like one got what he deserved." Wrong answer. Steve grabbed the guy and told him, "That guy is my brother, and he's dying, so you better give me another explanation." The owner spotted Steve's gun, which I believe was located quite close to his face, and discovered a more honest approach. "I thought you were lawyers. I wasn't even here." Jim was watching every face in the bar, waiting for someone to move, but nobody did. The same energy that carried the two of them in carried the two of them out. They went back to my in-laws cottage and sat down in the kitchen while the adrenalin proceeded to leave their bodies.

Jim recently told me that the chain of events—the drive back, walking in the bar, watching the faces as the place went silent, and, most of all, knowing the potential of what could have happened, and thank God for what didn't happen—is a day his memory will never be able to erase. Jim finished by saying, "You see what we did in the movies, and when it was over, you can't believe it happened. To see how that went down and to feel what I felt was indescribable."

Eventually, the two of them made their way to the local police station. That visit was a bit more relaxed. I think Jim just stayed in the car.

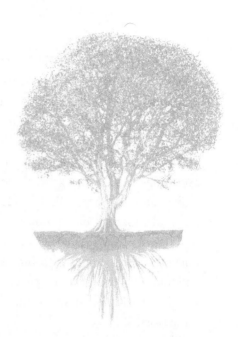

what now?

As I indicated before, UPS was my place of employment since I was twenty-three. At the time I was hired, I had one child and one on the way. UPS was heaven sent. I sincerely enjoyed every day there. Having been employed at a small family-owned company before I was hired at there, I was in awe of what it was like to work at a Fortune-500 company. I was making more money than I had ever dreamed of, and I was amazed at the opportunities the company provided every person who walked through the door. I could not have imagined working anywhere else.

Someone had to notify UPS of what had happened to me. That call was placed by Mary Beth to a manager I had become quite close to. His name was Thomas Farrell. Thomas was an Irish guy who took a liking to me and was the District Sales Manager for Chicago. I was set to be promoted to Sales Manager in a few weeks, so to say things were going good there for me would be an understatement. Mary Beth told them there had been an accident, and it didn't look good. After she explained to Thomas what happened and about my prognosis, he pulled those I worked with into a room, shut the door, and told them what had happened. He then put the other Chicago locations on speakerphone and told them the same story.

Thomas told me years later that this scene wasn't pretty; he said there were a lot of tears. UPS, as big as it was, still felt like a small company. Once you were a UPS employee, you were family, and to this day I thank that version of UPS for the support I received. My life felt like it had two pieces: UPS and everything else. You see, I was always the one they asked to *liven* things up, the one they depended on to break the ice, and back then I enjoyed that opportunity.

The clients I took care of were notified that there had been an accident, and their accounts would be temporarily, but most likely permanently, covered by someone else. I know I had made a lot of friends with the clients I was responsible for, which was my way of managing accounts. First, I would sell myself, which was easy. There wasn't anything special about me; I just tried to make my clients feel like they could trust me. Once I *sold* them on the fact that I would handle their account to the best of my abilities, I sold them on UPS. I always believed that you have to trust the person selling the product before you can trust the product. Sometime later, it was nice to be given the log of all the calls that came in daily from my clients who wanted to know how I was—one of those things you can't put a price on.

The hospital in Milwaukee was far from my suburban Chicago home, and it was hard for my family to travel there, especially Mary Beth, who had to take care of our kids. There was no improvement while I was in the Milwaukee hospital, and I was expected to stay there for a long time. To make it easier, Mary Beth arranged my transfer to a trauma center in Chicago. The doctors in Milwaukee thought it would be okay when it was first discussed, but when the day came to transfer me, I was not doing well and the doctors advised against it. After talking to the doctors and being told that she should look into long-term facilities for me, Mary Beth went ahead with the transfer. I was transferred again in a Special Care Ambulance to a trauma center in Chicago on November 27 and admitted to the neuro-critical care unit under the care of Dr. Synkowski.

Upon my initial examination in Chicago, Dr, Synkowski told Mary Beth that had he seen me immediately following the injury he would have recommended surgery to relieve the pressure within my skull caused by the swelling of my brain. However since it had been so long since the injury occurred, he would wait to see how I progressed.

I was given more cat scans and MRIs when I arrived to check for improvement. I was placed in the intensive care unit on the fourth floor—the floor for patients who have suffered strokes or brain injuries.

There was something about the amount of damage I had suffered that confused the doctors. It was not something that was very important to my treatment; however, I'm told it was brought up several times to family members. What was confusing to the doctors was the amount of damage suffered from a punch to the head. Not that a punch could not cause significant damage; but there was damage in areas other than where I was punched. It did not make sense. There we no abrasions on my face or forehead indicating my head had hit the pavement, which could cause additional damage. Keep in mind that my skull was fractured, and there were abrasions indicating blunt trauma on my head under my hair. The only visible signs of trauma were indicated by the fact that my head was swollen and my face was purple on one side from blood getting under the skin. Something just did not make sense about the injury. The doctors said that it was the type of damage caused by a severe beating.

My friends were allowed to visit me in the intensive care unit. Mary Beth would ask them to bring food that might trigger my desire to eat. She would tell them there was no guarantee I would be awake, but if I was, maybe food would activate something. They would bring

McDonald's hamburgers or pizza from my favorite parlor, DiGuido's Pizza back in Mount Greenwood. If this didn't get me to eat, nothing would. In those moments when I was awake, the nurses tried to feed me. I wouldn't eat a bite no matter how hard they tried. I had no desire to eat; basically, I was not aware that eating was even necessary. One thing I consistently asked for at both hospitals was Coke. I just wanted to drink Coke. Now, if that isn't a perfect commercial: *Coca-Cola, the soft drink those with brain injuries ask for first.* There was no change in my condition for several days.

No more than two people were allowed in the intensive care unit at one time. Mary Beth said she would catch my friends and family members talking to me, and it would break her heart to hear what they were saying.

Seeing me tied to a bed was hard to bear; however, the sight of friends and family leaning over me, trying to say anything that might make a difference, was very emotional. I was told how my brother John, who had to head back to work in Missouri had said good-bye to me, left the room, and a few minutes later came back, did it again, and then finally a third time. John had told me years later that he was sure that was to be the last time he saw me alive, and it was tough to leave.

There were times I would wake up and begin to scream two words: *"My back!"* This went on for days. The doctors assumed that something must have happened to my back or hips, so they ordered more X-rays. A little more radiation at that point couldn't hurt. It was determined through a series of tests that my brain had bled into my spinal column, which caused the nerves to go a bit haywire. That was the cause of my back pain, and I am sure it caused a few other issues.

One morning, my condition seemed to get progressively worse. It had been more than two weeks since the injury, and going into a deep coma at this time was not a good sign. I wouldn't respond to the sternum rubs or any attempts at stimulation. A cat scan revealed that the swelling in my brain had become worse. Dr. Synkowski came with a handful of X-rays while my wife, mother, and brother-in-law Mark were there with me. He called the three of them over to review the X-rays. Now the perception the doctor gave to the three of them was that he was going to provide some good news—not the case. As the X-rays were shown to all, he casually announced that he recommended removing part of the left front temporal lobe in order to relieve some of the pressure, so that the rest of the brain would not suffer additional damage.

My mother fainted and my brother-in-law Mark caught her before she hit the floor. As Mary Beth and Mark sat on the ground with my mom, the doctor explained the procedure. He wanted it to be done right away. My mother woke up and asked if I "would be like *One Flew over the Cuckoo's Nest?*" She really said that. You have to know my mom; this statement would not shock anyone who knows her. To this day, that still makes my brothers and me laugh.

Mary Beth initially said she would take me out of the hospital before she would let them remove part of my brain; however, the doctor explained her choices and the potential consequence of those choices. The doctor's belief was that I would die if this procedure was not carried out. If the operation were to take place, Mary Beth would have to sign the consent forms. She truly agonized over the decision. She wanted to know what the result of the surgery might be. Would it improve my outcome or would it make it worse? I am sure the thoughts she had were no different than those of others who had to face this same type of decision. One month earlier the most difficult decision Mary Beth had to face was where to go shopping. Now she had to decide whether to let them remove a portion of my brain. The resulting thought had to be, as it was in this case, *What type of person will he be if he survives this surgery?* They had no answer for her because there was no clear outcome: nobody ever knows.

The decision was made to re-evaluate my condition prior to surgery, which was scheduled for the following morning. If there was no improvement overnight, Mary Beth would sign the consent forms, and they would proceed with the surgery. Completely devastated and in total disbelief, Mary Beth said she ran to the ladies' room. She told me this was when the stress of all this had finally caught up with her; she said she just sat on the floor in the bathroom and cried.

five a.m. operation day

There appeared to be no change, so the consent forms were signed. My whole family was back by five; surgery was set for 6:30 that morning. My brothers had come back into town to see me before I went into surgery. I was given last rites...again. Upon entering the intensive care unit, Mary Beth had asked the nurse if it would be okay to try and wake me. "Absolutely," was her reply. Mary Beth walked over to my bed and began her attempt to wake me. After a few sternum rubs I became somewhat responsive, so she continued on with renewed hope. With every sternum rub she was whispering, "*Please, Bri, wake up, wake up!*" After a minute or two one eye had slowly opened up as Mary Beth said softly, "Hi, Brian," to which I quietly responded, "Hi, Mar. Can I go home now?"

Mary Beth turned toward the rest of my family and said excitedly, "I think he's better! I think he's better!" Moments later Dr. Synkowski entered the room and was greeted immediately by Mary Beth saying, "I think he's better!"

Walking over to my bed, Dr. Synkowski said, "Hi, Brian. My name is Dr. Synkowski. How are you doing?"

I'm told I said, "I think I have had better days," although I'm not sure if the words came out in that order. I then proceeded to say the names of those in the room I could see.

After observing my condition and at the urging of my family to figure out a way to delay this, Dr. Synkowski gave it some thought, looked around the room at all the faces, and said, "I think we can postpone this surgery." He went on to state that my progress would be monitored during the course of the day, and although surgery was still a possibility, this was a very good and most surprising turn of events. My family cried—every single person in the room cried. Mary Beth had that type of shock where you just don't know any other emotion except elation. Steve acted as though he just won a title fight, thrusting his arms in the air. Steve later told me that as he spoke to Dr. Synkowski, about six feet from me, they heard a faint voice singing Englebert Humperdink's *"Please Release Me, Let Me Go."* The doctor with his back to me asked Steve, "Is that who I think it is?"

Steve peered over the doctor's shoulder and responded with a tearful laugh, "Yeah it's him." The swelling had gone down somehow and there was some light at the end of the tunnel. For clarification purposes, I do not listen to Englebert Humperdink, but mean no offense to those of you who do. When Mary Beth tells the story of this particular event she still cries. Based on what I was told by those who were there, you had to see it to believe it.

The reason the swelling that nearly resulted in an operation had returned was leaked out to Mary Beth and my mother by a nurse who was making my bed. She had taken a few days off and was unaware of what had almost transpired. Here is how that went down: Mary Beth and my mom were on the side of the bed as she changed my dressings and made my bed, of course, with me still lying in it. She was talking to me in that *mom to a baby* tone, "Brian, don't push with your legs when I pull you up."

She then turned to Mary Beth and my mom and said, "Last time we were doing this, he pushed off the bed while we were pulling him up and his head slammed on the wall. We were so worried when that happened."

Obviously, she assumed that Mary Beth and my mom already knew, but she was mistaken. The two of them were in shock because I almost had part of my brain removed due to this, and had the doctor known it, he could have treated me for what it was. My mom was so upset that she ran over to the nurse's desk and pounded on the desk, screaming, "Why didn't you tell us you slammed my son's head on the wall? Where is the incident report!" Mom rarely gets upset; however, I guess I see her point on this one. What is absolutely strange to me is, of the few minutes of memory I have of the first three or four weeks, my head slamming off the wall was somehow stored in that small amount of memory. I guess coma or no coma, when your arms or legs are tied to a bed and you are temporarily untied, you get a bit squirmy. What I did was position my left leg for a push; the right leg was partially paralyzed, so the left would have to do. When the two of them pulled, I pushed. As I said, the result was a *head slam* off the wall. Now don't get me wrong about remembering this: what I remember is my leg pushing and the two of them pulling. That is the extent of it, and yes, the doctor was quite upset when he was approached by my family.

Rehabilitation would start right away. The swelling coupled with the injury had destroyed part of my brain. More specifically, the worst damage occurred to the front left temporal lobe, which controls emotions, memory, reasoning, and temper to name a few. I had lost forty pounds, had limited strength on my right side, limited balance, and triple vision in one eye. Physical therapy would be very interesting. I was totally uncooperative. First off, I had no clue where I was, what had happened to me, and was not aware that I was different. A phone was placed next to my bed when they put me in isolation with a twenty-four-hour nurse. With this phone, for example, I would call friends, explain that I was home, and ask them over to the house for a party. Mary Beth said it was common for me to call her at three in the morning. She said it was so often like a dream. I would start out sounding normal, then the conversation would just lead to questions like: "When are you coming to get me?" or, "Did you know I am in Mike's basement?" You see, I had my long-term memory, but no short term, so remembering phone numbers was not a problem. It was what might come out of my mouth, courtesy of my *brain in distress,* that created the problems.

Here is where the *phone* situation gets strange but somewhat comical. As I said, I had long-term memory but no short term, and since I had no idea what was going on, I made a few calls to my UPS customers. I remembered some of the numbers that I would call daily when at work. These customers were my larger clients. My time awake was minimal at first, so I guess I would become mildly alert for minutes at a time and do whatever the working parts of the brain decided to do. So here is what happened: UPS had made calls to all of my clients explaining what had happened, informing them that my accounts were being reassigned. From what I am told, at least three of those clients received a call a few weeks later from me. I guess I called and just started talking; about what, I do not know. These clients knew the content was *way out there,* though they were confused nonetheless, so they called UPS. Someone at UPS then called the hospital and Mary Beth to determine what was going on. Hospital officials told UPS that there was no way for me to understand what I was doing. It was agreed upon that the phone would be pulled away. They probably just unhooked it. I would have never known.

As therapy continued, I became increasingly more violent towards the hospital staff. I was scheduled to be at the Rehabilitation Institute of Chicago for six months. The R.I.C., as it is referred to, was located directly across from the hospital. As it appeared, I was not amused by the thought of rehabilitation. I really could not tell you why, since I have no idea what was trying to make its way through my mind; however, it appears that I was only aware of one version of me, and that version seemed just fine. I remember being strapped to a harness in an attempt to get the right side to catch up to the left; outside of that, my memory on the rehab side is blank.

While I was in the hospital, my brothers, Mike and John, set the Christmas tree up for Katie and Jimmy. The kids and I did it every year, always the day after Thanksgiving. My brothers said Katie told them as they were decorating the Christmas tree, "My dad is never coming home, is he? I know he is going to die, isn't he?"

Katie picked up on so much, and she knew something was way wrong. John said that he stared at Mike, each waiting for the other to say something. Finally, they both explained to Katie and Jimmy as best they could that one day I would be home. John said that in all his years of teaching, this was the hardest class.

Eventually, Mary Beth decided that it was time to bring the kids up to see their dad. They were nothing shy of completely excited. Both of them expected to run in the room and see their dad as they knew him, and in their minds there was no reason why they should not see exactly what they were expecting. I was tied to the bed, so that might have come off as strange; however, it was something that they would not immediately notice. I am told they ran to the side of the bed, and I just looked at them and said, "Hi," with no emotion, which took both of them by surprise. I am sure they wanted me to be as excited to see them as they were to see me. The reason for my emotionless response had nothing to do with not loving my children, and my normal reaction to seeing them was always excitement; however, I was not normal. In my mind I could not process when I had last seen them, what was going on, and that I was somehow different. The mood of my brain was constant frustration in those few moments I was awake. From what I am told, most times that I was awake I demanded a cab; maybe I was more concerned with getting that cab when they arrived. Please keep in mind, your brain is responsible for everything you do, say, think, and feel, and my brain was *not* working very well. I was like an eight-cylinder engine running on one cylinder, and when the rest were going to kick in was the question only time could answer. There is the chance you may be left with just six cylinders, and if that is the case, you learn to do the best you can under the circumstances. Your brain really has very little to work with, so you just have to take these and all the other situations in stride. My daughter, Katie, still remembers that visit.

The kids would draw pictures for their mom to tape over my bed and make recordings on their tape recorders for me to listen to. I just wasn't sure who they were or what was their role in my life. Although I never thought of it then, what role was I actually going to play in their life? To this day, Katie remembers the hospital visit as if it were yesterday. Of all the times of the year to get *mentally derailed*, why Christmas? This covered three holidays in a row, Thanksgiving, Christmas, and New Year's Eve: a trifecta.

I was ready to begin my rehab at the R.I.C., which was supposed to be step one. Everyone assumed the recovery stage was set. I was awake long enough to go along with the rehabilitation schedule; the threat of surgery had passed. All good, but all wrong. Day one lasted no longer than me being brought over there and then me fighting to leave. I'm told that my first and only day at the rehabilitation center went something like this: I walked in, looked around at all the patients, and proclaimed, "I do not belong here!" I'm told that I refused to cooperate. I was returned to the hospital. After being returned to the hospital, I again went off the deep end. I don't know the exact chain of events that transpired after I verbally and physically expressed my thoughts regarding rehabilitation; however, I managed to find the clothes I had on the night of the accident, put them on, grabbed my walking cane, and hobbled on down the hallway. I was leaving. Right on! I was a decision maker after only one day in rehab.

During this time, a call was placed to Mary Beth, and she was basically told, "He is all yours. We cannot control him. Please come and pick him up." The day Mary Beth received this call, she had just returned from Christmas shopping for the kids. She told me it was actually the first borderline normal day since the injury. Well, so much for normal. Mary Beth later told me that when she arrived at the hospital I was at the end of the hall leaning on my walking cane in the original clothes I had on the night I was injured in Wisconsin. I was cursing and threatening anyone who came near me. She pleaded with the nurses, "What am I supposed to do with him?"

"You have to take him home. He refuses to cooperate, so there is nothing we can do," they said. The security officer assisted Mary Beth in getting me to the car, and off we went. I actually remember part of the ride home. I remember lying in the front seat, which was reclined, looking over at Mary Beth driving the car and wondering, or just trying to remember how to operate a car. On the trip home, Mary Beth picked up Katie and Jimmy at my parents' house. Although they were only six and seven years old, after seeing me that one time during my hospitalization, they knew I was not the same person. They were just glad I was home, I think.

I don't recall much at all about the hospital stay, and judging by the hospital records I have read, I think that is a blessing. If the records are any indication of what limited thoughts my brain was thinking, anyone who works in that particular section of the hospital and deals with those who have any version of the type of injury I have should be given the Medal of Honor. I will tell you that my total memory of the three hospitals I was in prior to being released, or *evicted,* as I like to put it, totals about three minutes. I recall seeing my dad out of one eye as I was being shoved into a tube (MRI). I recall seeing my brother Mike sitting in a corner. I remember being hooked up to the body apparatus that was supposed to help me with walking. I also remember a hallway and a stairwell. I recall getting out of my bed after being placed in a room with a twenty-four-hour nurse. I don't remember what transpired, but I remember she was an African-American, and she was trying to stop me from doing whatever it was I was doing.

There is one small memory I have about my confinement to the room with the twenty-four-hour nurse. The memory consists of making my way into the bathroom, leaning on the sink, and staring at my face in the mirror. I do not have any idea what was going through my mind or what I was thinking at that time. I look back now and wonder if I noticed how thin my face had become, or if I recognized whom I was staring at in the mirror. All I remember is that brief moment. My next memory is being driven home.

When I did arrive home, I received assistance walking in the house from a neighbor who had been shoveling snow. He had seen the car pull up and noticed I was in the passenger side. From across the street, he saw Mary Beth struggling while she helped me out of the car. At that point the neighbor ran over and helped Mary Beth get me in the house. He held my arm and walked me to the couch. So there I was, staring at Mary Beth, the kids, and my neighbor. My neighbor kept saying, "You look good, Bri. You really do." I remember just sitting there with my coat still on, trying to absorb what was happening. It just felt surreal. I guess I wanted more than anything to be back home, yet when I arrived, it all seemed so strange. There was nothing I wanted to do. I couldn't go anywhere or really do anything, nor did I understand what I wanted to do. I just kind of existed. I imagine it was like bringing home a puppy from a shelter, a puppy that just could not be tamed and at any given minute could go completely overboard.

I remember leaning over and asking Katie to go get Dad's guitar. Katie ran downstairs and came back upstairs with my guitar and gently handed it to me. I kind of strummed it with the hand that was still partially paralyzed. Mary Beth said I stopped strumming after about ten seconds, handed it back to Katie with my left arm, and quietly said, "Well, I still suck at that." Years later, the wife of the neighbor who had helped get me into the house told Mary Beth that when her husband returned home, he cried when he described what he saw, telling his wife, "There is no way Brian will ever recover; he'll never be the same."

Home, a time of celebration...not even close. This is an extremely hard time for the ones taking care of a person with a Traumatic Brain Injury. Mary Beth wasn't given an instruction guide for taking care of someone with a TBI. There was nothing provided to her and no advice given when she had taken me home. It had to be extremely intimidating taking someone home whom the hospitals could not deal with. *Where do I take him for treatment? What is he going to do? What can I let him do and what is he not supposed to do? If he tries to do something he is not supposed to, how do I stop him?*

There were way too many questions with not enough answers. Mary Beth had no idea what to do, so she called Dr. Synkowski. He was never able to come to the phone, so she left him messages—a situation that can scare you. There is no telling what a TBI survivor will do or what he or she is thinking. Mary Beth had told my sister, Marilyn, about the phone calls with no response. Marilyn knew how desperate Mary Beth was, so she started calling the doctor as well. Finally, he called Mary Beth back, and he was not happy. First off, he started by voicing his opinion regarding my sister's messages. He assumed that Mary Beth had asked her to call, which was not the case. Mary Beth never knew she had called and told him that. She then began to explain to him that all she wanted was someone to point her in the right direction regarding what to do with me. She asked the doctor, "Where do

I take him for help? Is there another hospital that will take him?"

Finally, the doctor calmed down and said, "Take him to a local hospital and see if they can help." I believe there is more direction given to families now than there was then; as a matter of fact, I know there is. Either way, handing me or any TBI survivor off with no instructions can only result in a horrible experience. Mary Beth contacted Christ Hospital, located in Oak Lawn, Illinois, and my outpatient rehabilitation was arranged.

This is where the worst and hardest events to explain typically occur. You see, the assumption is, *Well, he's home, so he's okay.* Let me help you out: Yes, he is home, but he is the farthest thing from okay. This is the worst time. I was basically Forrest Gump and an extremely weak version of Rambo working together in an effort to escape the hell I began to realize I was in. My brain was on a carousel. Here is who could appear: the "Way too Nice" me, the "Extremely Quiet" me, the "Completely Unrealistic" me, the "One Trying too Hard to Prove I Was Normal," the "One Who Just Doesn't Understand Why Work Is Somewhere I Cannot Go," the "Car Is Something I Cannot Drive," and the "One Who Doesn't Have Any Clue Why I Have to Go to Therapy," and last but not least, the "One Who Goes Absolutely Berserk without Any Warning." This was the version that caused the most harm, and the version that is most difficult to talk about.

I remember falling to the ground and vomiting as my rage faded away. I know my brain struggled when this emotion came to the surface. The rage never lasted long; it just flared up and came right back down. Unlike the other emotions, this was the only one that had the aftereffect, which was falling to the ground and vomiting. The worst version of this rage came when I'm told I pinned Mary Beth to the ground and tried choking her as she begged seven-year-old Katie to dial 911. Katie vividly remembers that day. The majority of the time, when the temper took off, Mary Beth would run the kids out of the house, get into the car, and leave. I don't remember what I would do after they left, probably call someone on the phone, ramble on about nothing, hang up, and call the same person back, never realizing I had just hung up five minutes earlier.

Of course, I did not need to be at home to let the beast out. I do not remember what prompted this particular outbreak, but I do recall Mary Beth driving me somewhere, and because of circumstances that I could not control or understand, I snapped. We were in the car on one of the main streets near our house, and for some unknown reason I became enraged and got out of the vehicle when it came to a stop. I limped right through the four-lane highway, with her trailing close by. Eventually, I got back in, but this was just another one of the many hard-to-understand moments during that first year. There is no way to comprehend how bizarre an individual with a traumatic brain injury can appear. Those around you have no idea what you are going to do, what you are going to say, or when the next violent rage is going to happen. I should tell you that *anger* is not the only emotion I was capable of; actually, I was capable of displaying any emotion, and most often to the extreme. Anger is the one that seemed to cause problems. If I was *too nice* or *too depressed,* that really wouldn't have been an instant concern. Then there were the times when I would say or react to a situation or question in a manner that was reminiscent of the former me, and a huge ray of hope would run through the hearts of those around me. Personally, I had no idea which version of me was the former or the current.

Still not eating, all I wanted was Coca-Cola. Mary Beth said she had to show me how to eat food since I had no desire or understanding of food's purpose. Mary Beth said she tricked me into eating. How she worked this was pretty clever. Mary Beth placed a different food in front of me every day: hamburgers, hot dogs, sandwiches, pizza…no luck. She was just about to give up on getting me to eat when it dawned on her. She thought that since I would constantly ask, "Can I do this…? Can you drive me here…?" maybe she could plea bargain with me. So she tried, and I guess I went for it. A huge burrito was put in front of me, and she looked me in the face and said, "If you take a bite of this, I will take you for a ride in the car." I fell for it, and it was the first solid food in me since my injury. Now as I had not eaten in quite a while, it did not take much to fill me up. Mary Beth never did tell me if she gave me the ride in the car. Truth is, by the time I was finished eating what she gave me, I would have forgotten the original deal anyway.

I required "babysitters" when Mary Beth was not home, typically my friends. They would come over and just hang out, watching me like a kid. I'm not really sure I was even remotely aware that I was never left alone. I think I just thought my friends wanted to hang around. I was like a little kid who could not be left alone, a kid that at any moment could do or say something that would shock you.

As long as we are on the topic of being tricked, I should tell you about another normal activity I somehow did not remember—showering. Now it is not that I purposely did not want to do it; it is just that the activity, like eating, did not register. So how do you get me to shower? Easy: tell me someone is coming over to visit. That is how Mary Beth was able to get me in the shower. She would tell me: "Someone is coming over to visit, so we have to get you in the shower." She said it worked every time. It was funny how excited I would get when told that someone was coming to visit me. I really don't know if it was because I wanted to show whomever was coming over that I was fine or it was just something simple that made me happy. Well, happy enough to shower. When I look back now, I wonder if it was because I was like a kid at times, and by that I mean mentally. Having had children, I know there is that age where you do have to force or bribe them to eat and shower. I wonder if that was it, or I just lost track of those activities and was too busy trying to find my past through the blur of the present.

I wish I could tell you what makes sense and what doesn't make sense with brain injury recovery, but I can't. Yes, I guess part of my functioning brain knew something was wrong, but the damaged portion, I think, just thought it would be over…quick. As a general rule, I did not want to be babied; the reason was that I didn't see the extremity of what was wrong with me. One day some friends came over, and they were helping Mary Beth by watching me. They came down to the family room where I spent most of my initial awake time and just talked to me, about what I don't know. One of them who we called by his last name, "Frost," asked me if we had any cans of Coke and if he could have one. "Sure," I replied. "Let me get it for you."

He kept repeating, "No, Bri, no. I got it, just stay where you are." I didn't listen, grabbed my cane, and went to get it. He was right in front of me making sure I didn't fall. As we came to the stairs going to the kitchen, he jumped two stairs at a time. I wanted to do the same to prove I was as healthy as he was; no luck. I recall my right foot dragging on the first step, and there was no way I could do one normally, let alone jump two. At that moment something in my brain said, *You used to be able to do that,* and I had a moment of recognition that something was definitely wrong. He just got the drink himself. I will admit that if he wanted a Coke, he came to the right place. I'm sure there were cases of it, given that it was the only beverage I seemed to recognize.

I was taken to Christ Hospital for several types of therapy. I was to work on speech, occupational, physical, and cognitive skills. I was also monitored by a doctor who specialized in traumatic brain injury rehabilitation. Occupational and physical went okay; however, speech was strange, and the sentences would sometimes come out in a scattered order. The thing about therapy for brain injuries is that those responsible for treating you have no idea of what you were like prior to the trauma, and the sad part is, they just think that since you have a brain injury, you must be messed up.

While I was at Christ Hospital, I took a test designed for sixth graders to gauge my cognitive ability. I failed. This test result led to the rather strong recommendation that I spend some time at a cognitive rehab center called, go figure, Cognitive Rehabilitation Specialists. The one thing I did while in outpatient therapy was act, and I did it quite well. I tried as hard as I could to convince everyone who dealt with me that there was nothing wrong. That was easy for me, since I didn't have the ability to realize that there was a lot wrong with me. I remember the doctor in charge of my therapy would never look at me while he was talking about me. He would always talk to Mary Beth or whomever else was in the room, but never directly to me. It was as though I wasn't even there. I believe he pretty much thought I was a mess. This became something that most people did, unless he or she was asking me the most common question I received: "How are you doing today, Brian?" Every time someone would ask me that question, he or she would then turn to Mary Beth and ask, "How is he doing?" I could have just replied, "I am completely screwed up," and nobody would have heard me. My reply never really mattered. I am sure the only reason I was even asked that question, or any other question, was to see if I would reply.

Christmas came. It was held at my parents' house.

A typical Christmas, and lots of people stopped by to see who they thought was going to be the completely recovered Brian. Again, they all assumed that as long as you are no longer in the hospital, you must be fine. Every brain injury recipient would understand this shallow but somewhat universal view. A little bit of shock was in their Christmas stockings. They basically stared at me to see what I would do or say next. I was so different; when I first got there, I hooked up a video game to the TV so I could just keep myself amused and not talk to anyone. Regarding the video game, I played it quite a bit before my injury, most often with my son, Jim; however, I cannot tell you if anything I did there registered. I believe I hooked it up to avoid having to talk to those who were in attendance. Eventually, the quiet *Do Not Disturb* version went away, and I ventured downstairs. Before I made my debut, I had to sleep for a few minutes, and I remember my brother John waking me up when he arrived. I typically slept sixteen to twenty hours a day. John lived in Missouri, so I somehow remember viewing this as a sort of test, since he had not seen me in almost three weeks. I thought the look on his face might prove that I was okay. It was not the look I was hoping to see. At one point, and I absolutely do not know why this occurred, my guitar was handed to me so I could play and my daughter, Katie, could sing some Christmas songs. So they sat her next to me, and everyone gathered around, videotaping or picture snapping, or just plain staring. I looked up, and it was like some sort of strange event. I forgot what I was doing and just stopped, not to mention that I was still partially paralyzed on the right side, so I'm not really sure how that would have sounded. I think at first I wanted to prove that I could do it, and the more I tried to prove I was okay, the worse I appeared. Another bad dream you just can't wake up from.

When I was growing up, we would always attend Sunday mass. There was one thing Sunday mass was better at doing than any newspaper or town gossip, and that was letting you know whom in your neighborhood was sick or had passed away. You would always wonder if you were going to recognize the names when the priest read them aloud. Well, Mary Beth and the kids brought me to Christmas mass in our neighborhood church. Based on the minimal capacity my brain was functioning with at the time, I always wondered how it chose which memories to retain and which ones to let go. For what it is worth, the majority were let go. So here is one of the memories my brain chose to hang on to: We were sitting in Christmas mass when the priest read the names of those in the neighborhood who were very sick or had passed away. He mentioned one name that sounded somewhat familiar: mine. I remember slowly looking at Mary Beth after it had sunk in that the priest was talking about me. She just had this *I don't know* look on her face. I believe she did it on purpose so as not to confuse me. I am sure I thought the priest had to be mistaken, because that one-cylinder brain of mine thought I was just fine.

I recall a time after Christmas staring out the front window, watching my kids play in the snow. Leaning on my walking cane while dressed in my pajamas and a robe, I began to cry. I just remember thinking, *This thing is never going to leave.* Another problem was that I wasn't even sure what the thing was or how it got there. It really is impossible to describe what I was thinking, because the recovery progress is slow, very slow, and this type of feeling is very common in individuals with TBI. One other obstacle I had was the constant changes in personality coupled with an extremely moody brain. One minute my brain was handling the recovery quite well, and the next minute it was a train wreck.

Mary Beth was asked the same question by me every single day: "Am I doing better today than I was yesterday?" She gave the same reply every time: "Oh yeah, Brian, much better."

I know what you must be thinking by now; yes, I was at times a beast, but it wasn't really me. In a moment, my life, like that of every other brain injury survivor, changed dramatically. With a severe brain injury, I went from being independent to dependent, from being capable to incapable. What makes it worse is that I could not even remember it happening. I woke up and everything was different. What I did remember was what it was I used to be—independent, driving, doing things, and going to work. All of a sudden, people were telling me, "You can't do that! You can't get up and walk right now because you'll fall. No, you can't do this and no you can't do that." What do you think I was feeling then? Anger and frustration is understandable. People like me with traumatic brain injuries know what we want to do—we can see it—but most often we can't do it. I have said that I had no pity for myself; however, when I look back, I pity those who had to deal with me, specifically Mary Beth.

Fortunately, I now have the ability to understand why my family never wanted me to attempt anything without supervision. You see, several areas of my brain were affected, and the area most affected was the region that controls who you are—your personality. My ability to judge reality from non-reality; the ability to control my emotions and also my short-term memory were severely distorted. Those are just a few of the deficits that were clearly identified. In laymen's terms, I had no idea I was different and thought everything I did was normal. I had a lot more than just a brain hemorrhage; I also had several strokes and seizures that really took their toll on me. Sure, physically I was somewhat impaired; I just didn't have the ability to understand that these actually were impairments.

Looking back over this period, I basically experienced three different versions of myself: the first being me before I was injured, the second being the person I was after obtaining the ability to perform certain tasks, and the third, the person who finally, after my brain had begun to *rewire* itself, realized I was different and wanted more than anything to get as close to the original version as possible without anyone noticing something was wrong. Because the effects of my brain injury were more internal than external, I was able to get away with some of the plan—well, actually very little of the plan. Part of what causes society to misunderstand brain injuries is that they are, in most cases, internal. In other words, what society doesn't see, society doesn't understand.

Some of these moments can be frightening to those most often exposed to what is characterized as an individual having no control of emotions or, as society likes to put it, *a misfit*. However, some of these moments did produce a few lighthearted laughs at the expense of yours truly. Actually, I love hearing about those particular moments.

When you hear what went on with me by those who witnessed it firsthand, you may find it oddly amazing. When I watch and listen to my wife, kids, family members, and co-workers describe certain events, I find it truly amazing that the person being described is actually me.

One thing I was petrified to do after this happened, and still will not do it to this day, was place my hands on the crown of my head. I remember, for whatever reason, being scared to death because I was afraid my brain would growl like a stomach when it is hungry, and my hands would feel my brain making the noises. Yes, I know it is strange; however, there was nothing I could do about this fear. If you are wondering if I told the doctor about this, the answer is yes. There is a simple remedy for this, he said: "Do not put your hands there and you will be fine." You think I would have figured that out on my own. I guess that is why doctors make the big bucks.

I am not sure what Hollywood thinks, but from what little I have seen from it regarding brain injuries, they are sadly mistaken. You don't wake up smiling, hug everyone, and go home. I have seen *Regarding Henry* with Harrison

Ford. This is the only movie I know of that touches on the subject of traumatic brain injury. Although it was interesting at times, and the rehab scenes brought back some memories, viewers are left to assume that if you have one of these injuries, you will become the opposite of what you were. Harrison Ford's character is an arrogant lawyer who suffers a brain injury and comes back cute and deprived of intelligence. I am not saying that you can't be cute after suffering a brain injury; it just is not one of the adjectives the doctors use when describing what you may encounter as a brain injury survivor. They also don't use the words "lacking intelligence"; they substitute the word "impaired."

The hard part starts when you wake up. Early on in the recovery phase, you sleep all the time. It seems that you sleep twenty-three hours a day. I think when you are sleeping, that gives those close to you the opportunity to fantasize about the day you suddenly come out of it. The *calm before the storm* is actually the hospitalization period. Especially since, as a family member or friend, you can still dream the dream that he or she will wake up completely normal, give everyone a hug, pack up, and go home. There is always that standard book of lines told by the doctors, and my family, as well as the families of all others who go through this, have heard all of them. They typically begin with, "Would you sign the organ donor form?" and proceed from there. Basically, the family is told, in no certain order, "We don't know what he/she will be like if he/she survives." Mine were a bit more direct, the best being, "Make sure you pick a good nursing home." Other things said by doctors—keep in mind, I was in three hospitals—were: "He'll have no short-term memory, will not be able to perform any cognitive activities, may not walk, and he will never, ever return to work." Those by no means were all the things we were told. When you return home with nobody to care for you but the immediate family, welcome to hell. And I don't mean hell for the survivor. This was one reality TV show I am not sure you would want to watch.

One day Thomas, my division manager at UPS, came by the house. His purpose was to see how I was doing, present us with donations collected at work, and to talk to Mary Beth about my future. I was very excited to see Thomas; I recall being excited because I was going to prove how normal I really was, despite what the doctors had told UPS. Clear the way for the perfectly normal guy with a brain that was just shoved in a blender. Mary Beth said that when I finally made it up the four stairs to the kitchen and went to shake his hand, I missed and almost fell forward on my face. We all sat down to talk. Thomas then reached in his pocket and handed me a check. The check was the result of a collection that was taken up for us at work. I just placed it on the table like it was something of no relevance. The reason I did that was because it had no relevance to me, not at that time. I didn't recognize money or a check as something that mattered. Thomas recognized this and picked the check up and handed it to Mary Beth. Thomas began to talk, and Mary Beth said it was quite obvious that I had some issues. Thomas, after noticing that I really wasn't very good at digesting what he was saying, basically addressed his comments to her. After consulting with the doctors, UPS had decided to place me on *permanent disability*. In other words, there would be no return to work. Thomas assured Mary Beth that UPS would take care of my family. After they were finished talking, he gave me a hug and left. I wonder now if it is too late to take them up on the permanent disability. God knows there have been way too many days that specific thought stumbled through my mind only due to circumstances I cannot control, as well as the realization that I cannot do all that I used to.

In January, I was allowed to be by myself for several hours at a time. Mistake! I'm told there were times that I would stare out the window assuming, since Mary Beth was not home, that she would be returning soon, and if for some reason I felt she was purposely late or whatever, I would be the Rambo version, waiting at the door. Now picture this, I had lost forty pounds off my pre-accident weight of 165, was still partially paralyzed on the right side, one eye was closed from retina damage (I would see triple when I opened it), but there I was, and any strength left was ready to go. It was as close to having absolutely no control as a person could get. As quickly as the rage came, it left just as fast. What is strange is that I never knew what was going to set me off; there just seemed to be too many emotions trying to find their place in my head. Just a reminder, as angry as someone can get due to a brain injury that involves the left front temporal lobe, which controls emotions, you can also be on the extreme opposite of anger. Most often I was looking for reassurance that I was going to be okay, even though I wasn't sure what okay really was.

Being that I had no idea of what my body went through, I would be prompted to ask Mary Beth when things just didn't seem normal, at least for me. For example, being home alone was bizarre for me, even though I slept most of the time. One day something a bit strange happened. I was urinating, and blood coupled with blood clots were mixed in with the urine. Even I knew that was not right. So I called Mary Beth at work, and in a very quiet, almost childlike manner, I told her that I was urinating blood. She told me that when I was in my coma, I had removed all the monitors from my body. She said one of the things that I had removed was the catheter, and that was likely the cause of the blood clots. The removal of the catheter was by the famous first inmate to escape from the intensive care unit of the Milwaukee Hospital. I guess every bit of fame has its price.

That same January, a few friends came by to take me to Kevin Ashe's house. As you recall, I said earlier that I was doing some remodeling at his house prior to getting hurt and was on the last step, finishing the bar. Once we arrived, I looked around, trying to take it all in. I was excited about trying to finish what I had started months prior. The friends who had taken me over to Kevin's should have glued themselves to me. At first I could not remember the measurements I was taking. I would measure, go over to make a cut, go back and measure again, go over to make the cut, forget what I had measured, and head back again. Eventually, they would have me tell them what I measured so they could restate it when I got near the saw table. I recall the guys being nervous when I grabbed the tools. I am sure the saw felt like a million pounds due to the atrophy in my muscles and that my right side didn't have all its feeling back. Eventually, they left the room and let me do my thing. It could not have been more than a half-hour later and they were waking me up on the floor. The small amount of physical work, coupled with having my brain "work," had knocked me out. I finished what I needed to, and they drove me back home. The time needed to finish the work was minimal, maybe thirty minutes or so; however, I know I was brought over there in an effort to make me feel like something was still like it used to be. It was good to get out of the house and spend some time with those guys.

I eventually transferred from the hospital in Oak Lawn to a recommended rehabilitation center called Cognitive Rehabilitation Specialists (I was the poster boy there for years after I left—every kid's dream). Rehabilitation consisted of six-hour days, for one, sometimes two days a week, over most of the next year. I was not a model patient by any stretch of the imagination. I was mad at everyone, especially during the initial meeting, which included Mary Beth, the therapists, and, of course, yours truly.

As the therapist spoke, I recall thinking, *Me? Different? You people are the ones with problems.* I am positive that thought was transformed into words during the meeting. I likely added another week onto my sentence every time I spoke. In my mind, the only reason I was even attending this unnecessary rehabilitation was to prove to my family and doctors that there was absolutely nothing wrong with me. I recall sitting in rooms with the other patients and thinking, *What am I doing here?* and *Those people look like they are crazy.* I realize now that there were a lot of other patients there who, due to their deficits, had no idea they were different and probably wondered what they were doing there, and yes, I'm sure they thought I was crazy. I am not sure how to convey this, but I really had no idea that I was, for lack of better terms, different. That made the whole situation more bizarre and amazing at the same time. You know what a car is, you know what a television is, and you know to use the bathroom; you just haven't completely realized that someone who looks just like you has invaded your mind.

While at rehabilitation, the therapists taught me how to remember, organize, write letters, and work on the side (the right) where I lost strength. It was absolute torture! I would leave there crying every day, frustrated and angry. They would test the same things over and over. They would work on my memory, writing ability, planning, thinking, listening, and coordination. For example, in regards to planning, they would have me write out how I would plan a barbecue. Thank God I went there! The Cognitive Rehabilitation Specialists' plan was to have me manage while trying to work harder. I generally directed my frustration towards Mary Beth; why not? I seemed to blame her for everything else. What you need to remember is that I was the one with the injury, and she was the one with the burden. Virtually everything I described doing, whether it was being tied to a hospital bed, having fits, being taught how to walk with an uncooperative right side, Mary Beth was right there, standing next to me. Eighty percent of marriages in which a spouse suffers a TBI end in divorce. I do, unfortunately, understand why the marriage may end, as does Mary Beth.

It is somewhat ironic that I remember the memory rehabilitation exercises. The therapist would ask me for my St. Christopher medal, place it in a drawer, and tell me when the alarm they would set went off I had to ask for it back. At that point they would walk around the facility and touch things like the corner of a picture, and I would have to point to the exact same object at the exact same place. This seemed like a test to me, and I think I performed best at this. The rest of the testing was a blur, and from what I recall, I did not do very well. There were actually times when I would have to play with toys—toys that were initially designed for kids. These toys were the type where you would place round pegs in round holes. In case you are wondering, I think I did okay. The memory rehabilitation went on every week for most of the year, and I still call there with questions to this day. I guess I am an alumnus. My main focus was to get to the point where they would finally let me go back to UPS. I think they eventually let me return because they thought I might go insane asking every five minutes.

Driving was not something the doctors had covered, at least not to my knowledge. If they did prohibit it, it didn't matter, because I still had my old driver's license. At the time, I doubt they really put this at the top of their list of activities I should be able to do. I know the therapist at the rehabilitation center definitely covered it with my family. She said there was no way I was reasonable enough or rational enough to drive.

Another concern was the potential for seizures. I had plenty of them early on, and until your tests show no seizure activity in the brain, driving is a definite no. Being one who has loved cars since I was a kid, getting behind the wheel didn't appear to be off limits, at least it didn't to me. It wasn't something I initially wanted to do, but as my brain began to make minor strides toward healing, I guess the thought started to run through my scrambled head.

There was a day not soon after I was being left alone for short periods where I remember thinking, *Time to test the driving skills.* I remember taking the car out and driving around the neighborhood. Since my right eye saw virtually everything in triplicate, I stayed as far away from the curb on the passenger side as I could. I didn't go very far, just far enough to convince myself that I could drive. I couldn't wait to tell Mary Beth; however, she did not have the same enthusiasm for my ability to drive as I did. Today, the issue of driving is discussed with brain injury survivors and their families.

The chart below will give you an idea about the statistics regarding driving by victims of a TBI. This information was published in 1999, and there is not much information regarding driving prior to the late 1990's.

Percent Return to Driving			
	No	Partially	Yes
6 Months	69%	13%	19%
12 Months	60%	10%	30%

Data from ICRC Study, 1999

Someone once asked me if this incident brought me closer to the Lord. I replied, "It did not bring me closer, nor did it push me away." I did, however, say that had the Lord yelled *duck* on that November night, the basket passed at mass every Sunday may have been a little heavier.

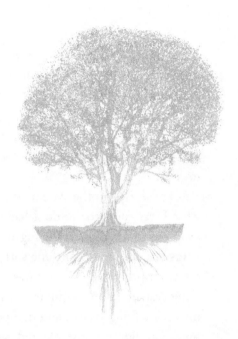

first steps

My doctors finally cleared me—after my begging—for a three-day, six-hour-a-day workweek. I still have the actual release form. I did every possible thing I could, and I am absolutely sure there may have been a few broken promises thrown in, to get the doctors to let me go back to the place with the brown trucks. Finally they caved, and in February 1993, after speaking with the doctors and therapists, UPS agreed to let me go back to work on the part-time basis outlined by the doctors. Mary Beth said the first two weeks I worked part-time, and after that

I was there full time, Monday through Friday. Unless I had to go to rehabilitation, which I did at least one day a week, I was at work. When I returned, I had no idea what I was supposed to do. I don't believe that anyone at UPS realized how complex brain injuries were, and since no one was holding me to the doctor's orders, I was on my own.

Let me explain the statement regarding not knowing what I was supposed to do. I had an idea of what I was supposed to do; it was organizing my mind to put the things I was responsible for in some sort of order. Picture this: my brain prior to the injury was a somewhat-organized filing system. After the injury, it was like someone took my brain's filing system and dumped it out on the floor. Sure, I could grab one file and remember what I used to do with that file; however, applying the information in a way that made sense was a severe struggle. I think the first few months were spent walking around trying to hide the fact that I was pretty much clueless. This was the beginning of my acting career. I realized quite quickly that even though a good portion of what I remembered regarding this job was located somewhere, I had to act like I was completely aware of what was going on. Either way, I was there. I struggled to recall names and procedures. It was not that I didn't know their names or faces; it was just getting the name from the inside of my brain to come out of my mouth. This is a truly bizarre feeling. I got in a habit of referring to everyone as *chief* or *buddy*. One day a person at UPS informed me that he was of Native American descent and took offense that I called him and others *chief.* Here I am with the IQ of a barbell, and he is trying to explain his Native American heritage to me. I guess I stuck with *buddy* as my *sorry, I can't recall your name* cover-up. To this day, I still use the same name, minus the -d and -y.

I wanted to go back to work because I assumed it would mean I was okay. Looking back, I think that just being at my place of employment was what I needed. I don't recall having any type of understanding of what I would to do once I got there. I am sure I was searching for a feeling of normalcy. I know now that there was no way I should have been allowed to return to work. There was another reason I felt that I had to go back to work at UPS. That reason, and most anyone who has worked at UPS will support this, was because you were always hesitant to call in sick. If you could make it to work, you didn't call-in sick. If you did call-in sick, there was always a guilty feeling. Our business was service. Pride in making sure we provided the best service was instilled in everyone who worked at UPS, so much so that calling in sick was avoided if possible. Now due to my limited mental capacity, I thought I was just fine, and at the same time my long-term memory was worried about not being at work. I had to go back. I do not want to imply that there was pressure on me to return to work; there was none. As I mentioned earlier, UPS had every intention of placing me on permanent disability.

A few weeks prior to my returning to work, I was driven downtown and given a promotion to Account Manager, which I was supposed to have received in December of

1992. The District Manager as well as my boss, Thomas, had similar thoughts on my pending promotion: "He's way ahead of what doctors predicted and to punish him by not promoting him would be a sin."

UPS was no different from any other company: it had no clue what a traumatic brain injury consisted of or what to expect. The truth is, the promotion was nothing more than an attempt to inflate some hope into me, and looking back I truly appreciate the reason my promotion was carried out. The comment made after I left the room was, "Just watch him for a while. If it doesn't work out,"—which they figured it wouldn't—"just put him on lifetime disability as originally planned." I believe I have since given them a pretty good perspective of what it is like dealing with, or trying to deal with, someone who has a brain injury. The chart below gives you an idea as to the chances of returning to work following a brain injury.

Employment Status					
	Student	Employed	Home	Retired	Unemployed
Onset	11%	57%	1%	11%	21%
6 Months	7%	17%	none	10%	67%
12 Months	7%	26%	none	8%	57%

Data from ICRC Study, 1999

National statistics show that within a year after a TBI, about twenty to thirty percent of people return to work.

That continues to improve with time. At twenty-four months it is up to about forty percent, but beyond that there is little change. Most people who get back to work after a severe TBI do so within two years of their injuries.

Not only does this information look at *if* individuals with a TBI return to work, but at the type of work they return to. Is it the same job they did prior to injury? If it is different? How different is it? The data show that the majority (over eighty percent) go back to the same job they had before. This is very important for Vocational Rehabilitation Services, because it indicates that the best approach is to return to the job they had, which is what happened in my case. Returning to work varies based on the severity of injury. Those with milder injuries return to work much more rapidly. However, at twenty-four months post-injury, about eighteen percent of TBI victims with milder injuries are still not back at work. At the same time point, about thirty-eight percent of those with moderate injuries and sixty percent of those with severe injuries are not back at work. Even those milder injuries have difficulties sometimes.

Keep in mind that my injury was a severe brain injury, and I somehow managed to get my clumsy feet back into the door on a part-time agreement basis after three months post-injury. I cannot believe I was in that building. I'll never know if it was a mistake or not. Looking back, the person that occupied my body had about twenty-five percent of the capabilities as the pre-injury version. The problem is that the twenty-five

percent I was working with was the basics, and that is all
that seemed to matter. The bottom line was, nobody knew
any better, and I guess I was difficult to deal with. If my
injury happened today, I would not have been allowed to
return. Also keep in mind, the original prognosis for me
after it was determined that I had potential for regaining
some of what I lost, was that I would be required to
attend a rehabilitation program for a minimum of six
months. The purpose of my initial rehabilitation was to
help me cope with my deficits and learn how to adjust to
life with a traumatic brain injury. It was not designed to
help me return to work. When I entered rehabilitation
there was no thought of me returning to work. Someone
give me an Oscar for convincing them to let me go back
to work…seriously.

The one thing the doctors had insisted on was that
I did not leave the building. The doctors were adamant
that any managing of accounts would be done over the
phone. The reasons were obvious; there is no way I
should have had face-to-face contact with any of UPS's
customers. On my second day back, however, I was on
my way to visit my first customer. Truthfully, with the
exception of one person who went to the library to get
an idea of what dealing with someone with a brain injury
was like, nobody at UPS had a clue. I was there full time
with the exception of the days I spent in rehabilitation.
An individual returning to work after a traumatic brain
injury should be monitored closely and have his or her
doctors' orders followed word for word. Not doing so
only sets the stage for disaster. You can perform some

basic activities and the perception becomes: *He's walking, suit seems a little big, and he's talking, so he seems okay to me.* There is no way on earth I should have been at work or driving, and absolutely no way I should have been placed in front of customers. But I was, and God only knows what I said to clients. I remember getting used to the idea that I needed to get really good at acting, because I didn't remember much of anything other than I was an employee of a trucking company called UPS.

The driving obsession, or the reality that I should not have been driving, was proven one day on the Illinois' tollway. At the time it was under construction, and cement barriers divided lanes, so you really had to have your wits about you when operating a car. One day I came out of the tollbooth and had to make a decision about which side of the barrier I should drive on. This is where the brain injury really reminds you it is there and would like to be recognized, because I could not decide which side to take, and the end result was plowing straight into the cement median. I was transported to a hospital for testing, and all appeared okay. However, I lost my car insurance. Here is a recommendation based on that occurrence: Never, ever mention to your insurance company that you had a brain injury and had a tough time deciding which way to go. Based on my experience, cancellation immediately follows your explanation.

Most of the people at UPS treated me very well. The fact that the doctor's orders were not followed was because nobody at UPS really understood what was going on and because I could, at times, appear normal. I stress the word *appear*. I would try to get through the job I was responsible for; however, I would often just end up falling asleep. I remember asking the doctor why I would fall asleep after trying to process or read paperwork, and his reply surprisingly made sense to me.

He said, "The part of your brain that processes that type of work has sustained significant damage; therefore, it has to work harder."

The result of my brain working harder was falling asleep. I would fall flat on my face at my desk—it was a classic crash and burn. Another area of concern that exists to this day was trying to stay focused during conversations or instructions. It was easier to play tennis blindfolded. I would start out listening, and in a flash whatever someone was saying to me was erased and replaced by whatever my brain decided to start thinking. It was the most frustrating, strangest thing you can imagine. No matter how hard I would try, nothing seemed to work. What I would do then, and still do now, was to start walking around the hallways, hoping to regain my damaged train of thought.

I spent so much time trying to figure out ways to speed up this time of frustration and get back to what I thought may have been a more normal time. What I learned then and still know to be true today is that I would cling to what I could still do well and try not to freak out over what I couldn't comprehend. Trying to absorb anything new was obviously not going to happen. To this day, I do believe that if I were asked what I most deserve, I would reply an Oscar for my acting efforts. If I had a gallon of gas for every time I said, "Absolutely. I know exactly what you mean," I would never have to stop at a gas station again…ever. Most times when something was being explained to me, I would be thinking, *I am not remembering one word of this.* I would just shake my head and try to let whoever was speaking think I understood every word that was said. What I did do, in the event someone was standing next to me while someone else was talking to me, was ask that person what was just said to me. I just didn't have the memory capacity. Initially I was told that I would never have a short-term memory at all; fortunately, this was not true. I did have some short-term memory at the time, but it was limited, very limited. So I would just act as if I understood every word being told to me. This capacity issue will be a problem for the rest of my life; I just have to continue to find ways to compensate. In a weird way, I got used to it, like I got used to the other deficits.

It still amazes me that one month after I returned to work, I was sent to a job training class for my new position. This school was in a suburb outside of Chicago, and I would be away for a week. Sending me to this training was way too much, way too soon. I remember showing up, and I didn't say a word. I was lost. I just stood there silently at the check-in. Mary Beth had driven me to the school and I remember panicking at the thought that I had forgotten to pack one of my medications. Fortunately, Mary Beth found it when she returned home and brought it back to the school. The school was held at Ronald McDonald University in Oak

Brook, Illinois, the campus McDonald's Restaurants use for their management training. Sleep was something I did as often as possible, as my brain needed a rest after any bit of cognitive work. That being the case, waking up was extremely difficult: so difficult that I had three alarms. The first was the clock radio, the second was the wake-up call the front office would provide, and the third was a co-worker who would bang on the door until he heard me say that I was awake. Most of the time it worked out pretty well.

One particular time when it did not work out was a bit of a nightmare—the result of my not having the capacity to use proper judgment as well as being too easily influenced. During this class, two of my fellow co-workers asked me to go out for something to eat. I had known them for years, so I agreed to go. After we had eaten, they wanted to go to a bar for a cocktail. I agreed to go; however, I told them that I could not have alcoholic beverages.

We arrived at the restaurant/bar, and it was a bit crowded and noisy. I ordered my Coke with ice and listened to the two of them, providing what input I could. After a few drinks, one of them suggested that a beer would not hurt me. I explained what I was warned about consuming alcohol and the dangers. However, I caved in and had almost three beers in a two- or three-hour period. I don't recall much that was unusual about the effects; of course, feeling unusual was something I had become accustomed to. That they thought I could have a beer was an honest opinion, and that I did have one was not their fault. You could have convinced me of anything at this time in my recovery. Chances are, I most likely wanted to have one only so that I would feel a bit closer to normal. Not that drinking was important, but I longed to do anything that was a normal part of life prior to my injury. We proceeded back to the school. I went to bed around midnight.

Sometime in the morning, I woke up on the bathroom floor with someone pounding on the door in an attempt to wake me. I felt extremely weak and totally confused. I had suffered a seizure during the night, and as the knocking ended, I had another one. After that last one I tried to crawl to the door. I never made it that far. Sometime during the morning I was able to get up, get showered, and headed down to class. I missed the class picture, but that seemed to go unnoticed. Without going into detail, there were a few times during that school where the euphoric me would show up and I would act totally irrational, so much that I recall that they brought in someone in to watch me and report back. I think the realization that brain injuries are not temporary was starting to sink in, and it appeared that the more exposure the folks at work had of me, the more obvious that reality became. All that aside, I never should have been at the school. It was like putting a five-year-old in the army.

There were a few instances that I believe were a bit funny, one of them being that I would lose most everything that came into my possession. If it was in my hand, I lost it. UPS eventually assigned someone to collect everything that my co-workers found. Most often items were found in the bathroom, cafeteria, or on the corner of someone's desk. An item that seemed to always disappear was the keys to my car, and I know now that I never should have been allowed to drive. However, I did, and the keys were an issue. On several occasions I found the keys in the car with the motor still running. Parking the car in the same location so I could find it seemed like a good idea; however, an even better idea was making sure I was looking at the keys in my hand as I shut the door, a rule I follow to this day. Another discovery I made was that carrying a wallet was definitely a bad idea. I realized this after about the tenth time I lost it. It just became obvious that the less I had to remember, or lose, the better. To this day I do not carry a wallet.

As my deficits became a bit more obvious, my manager, Thomas, asked to see my rehabilitation counselor. Two things were explained to Thomas: number one, watch me for extreme depression, and number two, be careful not to put me in situations that could cause my temper to erupt. Of course, the counselor had some input into the fact that they were letting me out of the building. It really did not make a difference what the counselor thought; I was not going to stop. Staying inside the building would have been hard on those around me; even I knew that.

I continued to tire quite easily, so I would hide and sleep in the bathroom or an empty room instead of at my desk. I figured nobody was paying attention, so any room was fair play. The storage room, bathroom, it didn't matter; when it was time, I crashed. I'm told my sense of humor, which was one of my dominant traits, was for the most part gone. This was not a good sign. There were days where I just existed. My therapy continued. My right side was pretty close to normal as far as control was concerned, although I was still weak and my energy level was nowhere near normal. The more I realized that there used to be a different version of me, and that it was nowhere in sight, the more it played on my emotions, specifically depression and anger.

There was this one day when I guess I just seemed to be a walking zombie. Thomas had been cautioned to watch for this—not sure of the correct term, I'll just call it "walking body." Anyways, he walked up, tapped me on the shoulder, and pointed me into his office. Once Thomas got my attention, he asked me why I had been walking the halls. He was being very nice about it, like he knew what was coming. I cried non-stop. Truth was, I was scared. I knew I was a fraction of who I was, and there had to be more to life than this. I didn't say anything; he called the rehab facility, and I was gone.

There is this part of you that remembers the former version and becomes aware of the current and can identify the huge gap. This continues to develop, and the end result is not good. It makes you more depressed, and at times you want to give up. I realized they all knew how different I was; they had to see it or hear it. I kept thinking I was going to get over it. I stuck with what I could do best, and that was minimal. It was a good sign that I was starting to question what skills were left. That I knew something was wrong was, in my opinion, the only way I was going to make progress.

To this day I wonder what people who had spent time near me at work, or anywhere else for that matter, thought. I always try to remember what it initially felt like to try to fit in. It was so strange. The problem is, your brain is like a radio; your emotions are like different stations on the radio, and you have no control of what station is going to be tuned-in next. It still applies to this day; I just learned to live with it.

Just to give you an idea of how strange things can be for a TBI survivor, especially the first year, the following is a story recently told to me by someone I had worked with before my injury and for years after my injury. His name was Ray, but I used to call him Senator Ray because he looked like a senator, and if he wanted to, he could convince you that he actually was a senator. Ray described a time during my first few months back at work where I just walked up to him while he was having a conversation with another co-worker and started rambling. No *excuse me* or explanation for what I had to say, I just started talking. Ray told me that what was startling to both him and the individual he had been speaking with was that I kept referring to him as someone else, repeatedly calling him by another name. The conversation I was having with Ray was actually a subject that had nothing to do with him, but rather everything to do with whomever it was I believed I was talking to at that particular time. Ray said he was finally able to get me to stop, and very eloquently he explained to me that he was Ray and not the person I imagined him to be. Now I had known Ray for years, so I have no idea what was going on with me at that particular moment. Ray said that after he told me, I just stared at him, obviously confused, and eventually walked away. Ray said the co-worker who heard the whole conversation had one word: Wow! I asked Ray why he waited so long to tell me that story. His response was, "I never thought it was something you would have wanted to know until now." The range of where your struggling brain can take you is endless.

As I mentioned earlier, things just *pop up*, which are a result of a time I don't recall. When my brain was bleeding, which it did quite a bit, and due to the protective lining around the brain being torn, the blood moved where it could. One of the two places it went was into my eyes. By that I mean *behind* my eyes, specifically the retinas. I had always felt pressure in my eyes after my TBI, but nothing registered in my mind, so I am sure I just pushed it off as part of life. One day blood started coming out of my left eye, near the tear duct. I am sure I thought, *What did I pull out of there when I went a little haywire in the Milwaukee trauma center?* I called Mary Beth; she called the hospital, and I was in right away. Both my eyes were examined, and it was determined I had significant damage to the eyes. My vision was fine, it was just damage to the eyes themselves. The reason was that the blood had damaged the eyes, leaving scar tissue. Another side effect to this was that my left eye did not dilate. A side effect, which caused the pressure, was the swollen eye. One recommendation was that the doctors go in behind the eyes and try to cleanse the retinas. This was left up to me, and the answer was, for lack of better terms, a no-brainer...*no!*

I called Mary Beth in a panic. "They want to take my eyes out. The doctors want to take my eyes out!" I said. She calmed me down and assured me that they were going to stay right where they were. The remedy for this was steroid drops and an eye patch. I had to take the drops for two years in both eyes. The right eye acted up not long after the left eye. Unfortunately, this was only the beginning of the leftover effects.

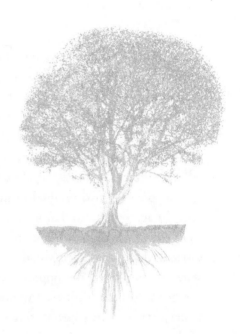

trial time and recovery

Things were heating up back in Wisconsin. A pre-trial was set in March, 1993 to determine if charges would be pursued by the state. I was not in attendance. My friends and one brother, Steve, were there for questioning. When Steve was told who the perpetrator was, he went a bit haywire and had to be restrained. I had no animosity toward Nick Smith, mainly because I had no memory of the incident, and I was more interested in recovering and moving on. I really didn't want to waste any time thinking about this, because there was nothing I could add to the topic. I could tell them everything I remembered until I put my jacket on to leave the bar. To be honest, what I do remember of the man who put me in this condition was little. I truly waited for a call from someone who would tell me to forget about the legal side.

The pre-trial had resulted in multiple charges being brought against Smith. For his attack on me, Smith was charged with assault with intent to do bodily harm. The assistant district attorney would be the prosecutor for the state. I was offered the opportunity to press additional charges as well, but refused. I wanted nothing more than to delete that future court hearing from my life. I thought of the pending trial, whenever it was going to be, and it gave me nothing but stress. I did not want to talk about it with anyone. I was driven up to Wisconsin to meet the prosecutor, but it was obvious there was nothing I could, or would, add.

Sometime in February, almost four months after my injury, I asked Mary Beth if we could go to the bowling alley. I had been in bowling leagues for the previous six years. Our team consisted of my brother Mike, Dad, and a few other friends. She said sure, so we headed up there. I grabbed my ball on the way out. I always dressed in a typical Chicago outfit: jeans and a t-shirt with some sports team logo. For a time after my little brain rattling, I seemed to forget about "fashion." That night I showed up in baggy sweats—I was still missing about twenty-five pounds—a sweatshirt, and hat. I was hoping no one knew where I had been. I wasn't ten feet into the place when someone from the league decided to welcome me back using the building's audio loudspeaker.

"Can I have your attention: we would like to welcome Brian Sweeney back from his near-fatal head injury." How nice is that, *welcome back from your head injury*. Looking back, it was somewhat funny how I was welcomed back with a nice gesture from the boys. However, it only took me about ten seconds to convince them that I was certainly not *back*. Anyway, I told my brother Mike, "I'm bowling." He looked at my dad and just went with the flow. You see, there was no—zero, nada—reasoning with me. So after all the other bowlers were finished welcoming me back, we started. First shot, *bam*, I fell right on my face. I got up slowly and acted as if nothing had happened. By the end of the second game, you would have thought I had run a marathon. Encouraged to sit down, I refused. This type of behavior was typical of me after the injury.

I had a plan to regain more of my lost physical ability. I guess bowling wasn't enough. I wanted to run again, and I wanted to be able to do it by March. Every time I would try, I'd fall after a couple of steps, simply because my balance had not caught up with my desire. This would only leave me more determined. To use this as an example, what happens during recovery is that you begin to recall things you used to do with ease, and you want to do them again at any cost. I was obsessed with regaining what were once my normal activities, like running.

Sometime in March I did run, not very fast, but I would consider it running. I was really excited. It was at night after a March snow. The street was clean, and I went for it. Not much speed, but I ran the whole block (okay, half) in a T-shirt, and I remember looking around as if I expected the whole neighborhood to clap—but nothing. If anything, they were most likely trying to identify the nut in the T-shirt running in the snow. You mentally keep a checklist of things you were not supposed to be able to do, but then did. For me, it gave me hope and encouragement. Sometimes when you fail it is discouraging, but you either fight or give up. I was not going to give up.

I had a plan to beat whatever it was I was going through. It is so difficult to explain what I was thinking because the organ that did the thinking was damaged and working overtime trying figure out new ways to do things. Looking back, I never thought or believed there would be anything permanent about whatever was the cause of all this special treatment. It will forever amaze me that I was so different and challenged, but most often never had the ability to realize it. I just figured I was going to fix it on my own. I imagine that many TBI survivors experience their recovery in the same way.

Let me give you an example. I knew my balance was not normal; I knew there once was a time when I could look up and not fall down. After my injury, if I looked at the ceiling—down I went. If I got up too fast, I went down. I knew that I should be able to run without falling to the left or right. So here was my plan at the time. I remember thinking, *How can I fix the balance issue?* I constantly thought that if I just fixed all the little problems, the big ones would disappear. Keep in mind, I was not dealing with a fully functioning brain. The plan was to sign up for a karate class and learn how to get my balance back. I'm just glad ballet didn't come to mind. I went to a karate studio, and I explained what happened to me and asked the instructor if he could help with my balance and coordination. His reply was, "Absolutely, we can help you." The next question he asked me was if I would like to get my balance back with cash or credit.

I signed up, and nobody knew I was taking karate lessons. I would say that I was going to a gym to do exercises that would help my balance, but instead I would go to the karate studio. I took lessons for two months, and I don't have a clue if it solved anything. I am quite sure that at the time, in my mind, it did solve something. Most likely it was simply time that helped my balance, but I remember thinking I was getting smart for developing the idea. I thought about so many ways to fix the brain injury thing. There was no way to stop me, and reasoning with someone with a recent brain injury is as close to the impossible dream as you will ever get. Looking back, I cannot believe I actually signed up for the class, and better yet, somebody actually allowed me into the class.

The old me was starting to show up a bit more often. However, the depression, migraines, and my attention span being the length of a commercial, were becoming a way of life. I think this was the time when my conversations would really start to raise an eyebrow. I was starting to look more like myself, and on occasion act like my old self, so people thought that I must have been okay.

Not that you want to be different; it is just that the more normal you appear, the less tolerant those you interact with become in regards to your shortfalls. All any brain injury survivor wants is a bit of understanding—period, end of sentence.

Therapy ended in June 1993, but resumed in July. The depression had been a burden I couldn't shake. I cried at work after not knowing what to do. I had become violently angry towards those who would, in my opinion, treat me as though I were "less than I was before." At times I had no desire to exist, and I couldn't understand it. The obvious defects were becoming more apparent as I began to understand what really had happened. I was afraid that I would always be labeled as *brain damaged*.

By June, I was doing better physically. I put fifteen pounds back on and could run fairly well. My brother Mike asked me if I could build or assist in building a deck on his house. Being asked to do things like this was a nice feeling, since for the most part I never received requests to do the things I used to do, and after a while you start to realize something is missing. Actually, a lot was missing; however, little pieces of the puzzle tended to fall in place over time. This was likely the first time that I became conscious of the deficits I was struggling with, as well as my inability to stay focused and control my temper. What happened was typical if you were living in my house, but not very typical if your exposure to me was nothing more than a quick visit to hear me say *hi* and answer *fine* to your typical *how are you feeling* question. Anyways, I was working on the deck with my dad, who, keep in mind, had

had a stroke the year before, so he and I together made a nice combination, along with my brother Mike and a friend. In the middle of working on the deck, I suddenly left to get my tires changed. No rhyme or reason; the impulse just happened to run through my brain, so I got up and had them changed. That I just stopped what I was doing and began to do something else was common for me. I have struggled to control impulsiveness since my injury. If the thought of something, anything, enters my head, chances are I stop what I am doing and go in the direction my brain takes me.

When I came back, my power saw had been broken. I tried to use it and became infuriated—not mad— infuriated. Mike told me years later that I grabbed a board and swung it at all three of them. I dropped the board went home and slept for hours. I came back later, and we eventually finished the job.

There were bright spots, or at least what I considered bright spots. My family was initially told by many doctors, at multiple hospitals, what their prognosis of my recovery looked like. I guess every shift doctor gave his or her opinion. Again, in no specific order, my family was told that I could be in a wheelchair for life, I may possibly be in a nursing home for life, and I may never walk or do anything physical. Also added to the list was the possibility that I may have limited, if any real cognitive skills, I would have no short-term memory, I may never hold a job, I would have migraine headaches and seizures for life, I would have minimal or no control of my temper, I could have vision problems, and my favorite, I could be *a vegetable for life*. I don't like vegetables, so I was not going to let this brain injury turn me into one. The bright spots were doing anything the doctors said I would never or could never do. Some other bright spots were getting rid of the after effects, such as seizures, for example. I had plenty of them the first month, so I was on seizure medicine, among other medications. During the summer of '93, I had tests performed on seizure activity. The doctors were shocked; the test revealed no significant danger of seizures.

That result gave me such a great feeling. The weird part was, I wanted to find out which doctor said I would have seizures for life and let him or her know that the diagnosis was wrong. The truth is the doctors were not wrong, they were just telling me what the test had revealed. I just was lucky with the results. I could (and would) still have seizures; however, the test had shown my chances were minimal.

Another test I took was an annual physical that UPS required of all management personnel. The year prior, I was told by the physician conducting the physical that I had completed the most sit-ups of all who were tested. I always tried to stay in the best shape I possibly could, so being told that was rewarding. I was looking forward to this physical. I was always hoping that somebody would tell me I was as good at something after the injury as I was before, or maybe even better. When I arrived at Luke Presbyterian Hospital in Chicago, I was happy to see that it was the same doctor who conducted my examination the year before. I had my workout gear on and was ready to do the physical part (push-ups/sit-ups) of the examination. The physician reviewed my chart and seemed to be in shock. I know I was still much lighter than the year before, but I figured I was "good to go." The physician asked me to please stay seated while he left the room. I heard him in the hallway talking to the trainer who was going to conduct the endurance or physical part. The physician said, "Don't bother putting him through any of these tests; he should be dead." I was floored. They both came back in and told me the tests weren't necessary due to all I had been through and was still recovering from. I demanded that they put me through the same tests as last year and what every normal person does. I tried so hard to beat my scores, going as fast as I could with the sit-ups, but fell short of the prior year. Looking back, I truly believe it was just another attempt by my recovering brain to prove that I was still the same. The good news was, I didn't have much body fat, which, of course, was because I had lost so much weight and had not yet developed a strong desire to consume food. This is not a recommended way of losing weight. (I am sure that you already came to that conclusion.)

Other bright spots were the result of my exercising bad judgment and by having enough of the *old me* left to convince others that I could do what they had been told I could not. Here is how one of those events went down. My brother-in-law Jon had a softball team that played on Sundays. Now softball was never that important to me; however, since I was told that I would most likely never be able to do this type of activity, it suddenly became important. I asked Jon if I could play on his team. I knew I still had balance issues, though they were nowhere near as bad as they once were, and it posed a risk of getting hurt, but I wanted to do it. I remember that Jon said, "The team is already assembled, but you can come out, and if I need you, you'll go in." That was fine with me. I asked him not to tell anyone what had happened to me. We were in the second game into the season, and Jon said, "You're going to bat this inning." That made my hands sweat and it still does just thinking about what it meant to me.

I had some practice swings before the game, so I knew I had some timing for hitting. I also figured out before the game that if I looked up to catch a fly ball, I would most often fall, so playing the outfield was out of the question. There I was, standing in the batter's box. Just standing there felt good. Here came the pitch. I was planning to swing before he ever threw it; I figured it would help my chances. It worked, or something worked because the ball took off down the third baseline and past the third baseman.

Jon was coaching first, and I believe he was as excited as I was since he had watched me go through the whole mess. I stumbled coming out of the batter's box as it was the first time since the accident I had to sprint; it actually felt strange. My legs had decent timing, but not yet near where I was hoping. When I reached first, I smiled. As I got settled at first, Jon gave me a pat on the back and said, "Proud of you, Sweeney."

That hit was really all I needed to place another check

in the "list of things I would never do again" box. I believe my desire to play was to confirm that I could still do the things I used to do. I'm pretty sure that based on my personality make-up, giving me a list of *things I should not do or cannot do* was similar to giving me a list of "things to do." I'm not sure if there were any more hits, and it didn't matter; I got the one that meant the most to me.

As much as I know playing softball was dangerous, even though it was limited, that was such a great feeling. I marked down those types of successes as major steps for me. Even I realized that it was more *above-the-neck* problems I was going to have issues with as the future became the present. By the way, my family never came to watch some of the events in which I participated, and I completely understand now. The reason was obvious; they did not want to see what happened when the risk was realized.

I have to give them credit; dealing with a TBI survivor in the initial phases of his injury is truly exhausting. The issue was trying to stop me from doing whatever I was determined to do. This was a serious dilemma, and it was not going to get better. I was kind of like a remote-control car with a broken steering mechanism. Sure, I would go the minute I had the energy; however, you just couldn't control which direction I was going. I couldn't even control which direction I was going. Makes you want to wear a helmet for the rest of your life, doesn't it?

In August 1993 I was back in Wisconsin where I was scheduled to be the star witness in Nick Smith's trial. This was the last thing on earth I wanted to do and dreaded every minute of it. What was I supposed to say? I didn't remember a thing, not sure it would solve anything, and the stress was definitely not doing me any good. It was strange, but Joe, Kevin, Henry, Tim, and I never talked about the trial before it took place. We also never spoke about the night I was injured before the trial, and for the most part we never spoke about it afterwards. Sure, I would get them to say something once in a while, but for the most part, if the topic was raised by anyone, it was dropped immediately. I always wanted them to talk about it, I wanted to know what had happened, but they just never wanted to discuss it. It was a significant piece of my life that was missing, and I wanted to know what happened. I know it bothered them, though there was never a reason it should have. It just happened and there was nothing anyone could do about it.

Trial time. The trial, which was to last three days, was being held in Walworth County, Wisconsin, and the local town was not very large by population standards, so it was a big deal. For months I was referred to in the area newspapers as the *mystery coma man from Illinois*, so these folks were waiting to see the rough and tough guys from Chicago. They were a bit disappointed; we didn't look too rough and tough. I have to admit, it was like going to court for a dream you once had; it truly was like a dream, a nightmare. A few weeks prior to the trial, I had requested to have a private meeting with Mr. Smith. I just wanted to hear him say something to the effect that he was sorry. If he would have apologized, I would have told the district attorney to call off the trial. My request was refused; there would be no meeting.

The courtroom was packed; there were reporters, the whole deal. I was not ready, but I thought this might close it out and I would magically get better. Not quite. My wife pointed to Smith and said, "There he is." Remember, she knew him from spending her summers in Wisconsin. He recognized her and seemed a bit shocked. I didn't remember a thing from that life-altering night, at least as far as what I assumed they would be asking me. I kept hoping Smith would come over and say that he was sorry; to me that would have been all I needed. My friends and I, my parents, my brother Steve, and Mary Beth just stood and stared. We were not allowed to enter the courtroom since we would be testifying. I was the first one called. Before I went in, I looked at Kevin, Henry, Tim, and Joe. I think we all wanted to run out the door; as a matter of fact, I know we did.

It was quite strange realizing that I was going into a courtroom to be questioned about something I could not possibly remember. I walked in with Smith staring at me. He had an extremely cold look; he most likely wasn't too thrilled about being there either. It was one of the strangest feelings I had ever experienced. There I was, recovering from traumatic brain injury, on the witness stand for something I had no memory of. I never, ever wanted pity, but I thought somebody should step in and stop this mess. I told the judge, the defense lawyer, the jury, and everyone in the packed courtroom that questioning me for something I did not remember was pointless. Now if you would like to question me about the life I had prior to this pointless, alcohol-fueled assault, I would be glad to answer those questions.

Kevin, Joe, Tim, Henry, and Steve were also called to testify. Tim and Henry cried on the stand when they were asked to recall the events surrounding the assault. Joe was still angry about what had happened, and that was obvious during his stint on the stand.

Kevin was nervous. They had a diagram of the parking lot and the bar in the courtroom. Kevin was questioned as to our location in the bar, the car's location in the lot, the location of the fight, and finally exactly how many beers and/or shots we consumed. The beer answer was standard: eight. Coincidentally, each of us answered eight. When they asked Kevin if we had ordered shots, he answered yes.

"What kind?" the defense lawyer asked Kevin. Turning red as a tomato, Kevin finally said, "Um, uh, Sex on the Beach." It was the only time I saw anyone in the courtroom chuckle, including the judge.

Steve went up with his police uniform on and described what he had experienced in his eight years as a police officer and how it compared to seeing me for the first time. Steve had told the jury and those in the courtroom how difficult it was to walk into an intensive care unit and see your little brother hooked up to systems designed to prolong his life. Steve told them how my face was purple due to blood under my skin. He continued by saying how hard it was to hear the word *vegetable* attached to his younger brother who had always been so full of life and the father of two small children.

Three days of testimony. The defense attorney tried to portray us as Chicago hoodlums. No luck. All you had to do was look at us and that accusation held no merit. We were just five boyhood friends trying to enjoy a weekend in a resort town, where a traffic accident made headline news, and *bam!* it happened. After testifying, the boys went home. The only ones left were my parents, Mary Beth, and me. We were treated to some of Smith's more intelligent friends. A few of them sat behind Mary Beth and me and would whisper, "You drunk, you just fell on your face." Comments directed at Mary Beth's were more to the tune of, "Hey, pretty lady, you with this loser?" She grabbed my arm and whispered to ignore it. I had more anger toward those two losers than the one who caused my injury.

It was very interesting for me, listening to all those witnesses testify about what had happened, who did what, and what I was like. At one point, the defense called a doctor to the witness stand to talk about the injuries that Smith had sustained. Even in my limited mental state, I had thought that was a bit odd to compare his injuries to mine. Actually, it was not even a comparison. Smith's attorney asked the doctor to describe what injuries he had sustained as a result of the employees and patrons beating him. I'm not sure why this was relevant since I had nothing to do with his beating.

When that brief moment in time was over, the prosecutor for the state asked the doctor to comment on my injuries. The defense attorney had a fit when the prosecutor asked the doctor to remain on the stand. The defense attorney demanded a mistrial. The judge told him the prosecutor's questioning was sustained and denied his request for a mistrial. The prosecutor asked the doctor to comment on what a person would or could be like if he had sustained the following: a subdural brain hemorrhage, lacerations to the brain, excessive bleeding to the brain, swelling of the brain, significant damage to the left frontal lobe, as well as bleeding into the spinal column. When the prosecutor was finished listing some, not even all of my injuries, he asked the doctor, "Could one or more of these cause death or permanent disability?" The doctor replied sternly, "Yes, definitely."

Bringing in a doctor to comment on the injuries Smith had received backfired on the defense. The injuries he received paled in comparison to mine. When the doctor was describing the injuries I sustained, the members of the jury looked at me with amazement.

The trial shed light on one fact: there were a lot of people whose actions led to my condition. First of all, the doormen were paid in drinks for working and were admittedly intoxicated. The patrons who had joined the employees in their beating of Smith were also intoxicated. His injuries were a fractured cheekbone and a sore back. I thought, *Had sober, reasonable people from the beginning handled this, none of it would have happened.* I never blamed anyone. It was a combination of alcohol and bad judgment. Unfortunately, I had nothing to do with why they beat him, but I paid the price for their actions.

The jury exited the court to decide the verdict. The room was silent; left from *my team* were Mary Beth, my mom and dad, and yours truly. The prosecutor came over to us and said that it would be in the best interest if the four of us would leave before the verdict was read. The concern was that violence might be the result of a guilty verdict, and due to the number of people on Smith's side, and knowing the harassment they had given my wife and me the day before, he strongly suggested we leave town. We took his advice and left prior to the verdict being read.

Nick Smith was found guilty of assault and battery with intent to do bodily harm. Sentencing was set for November 12, 1993, almost a year to the date of the incident.

Between the trial and the sentencing, I continued to slowly improve. My temper was a little more under control. Frustration was a major cause for my temper to flare out of control, and the first year was full of situations I couldn't manage. My short-term memory was still bad, but I laughed a little more. There are a wide variety of strange occurrences that accompany brain injuries. Some leave with time; others decide to stay. For example, I was still having, at any given time, multiple emotions running through my brain within a thirty-minute time frame. Fortunately, I realized with time that this maze of emotions was most likely temporary, so keeping them contained is an art I have become quite good at. I was no longer on brain seizure medicine, at least for the moment, so things were progressing. Life was moving on.

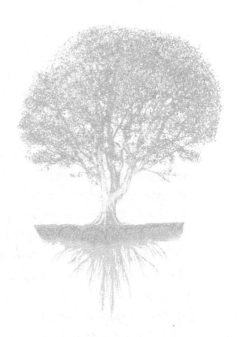

sentencing

I had dreaded this day for months, or at least since I had learned that there was no way the whole court mess could be avoided. I kept wondering what would happen if Nick Smith went to jail. Would he have a personal vendetta against my kids or me? Before the trial, we had been getting calls at home; the caller would hang up the second the phone was answered. This was before caller ID.

I had a dream, the only one I recall regarding this situation, and in that dream I was back in Wisconsin sitting on the dock that I had built near the house. As

I was sitting there on the end of the dock, I heard this noise and I begin to turn around when *bam!* a baseball bat smashes the back of my head. I remember waking up with ringing in my head—go figure. I think what made me worry at the time was that one significant blow to the head could kill me due to the damage I had sustained, so I was always worried about that—well, most of the time I was worried. I kept worrying about my family staring at his family and vice-versa during sentencing, and I just did not want to have anything to do with it.

The day before the sentencing, my brother Steve had driven up from Carbondale, Illinois, to attend. My friends, as well as my wife, were ready to go. I wasn't. I told them I wasn't going. I just wanted to end it and had been in distress over this day for too long. They were not very happy when I went to work that morning. I recall telling Thomas, my manager at UPS, that I was not going to go to Wisconsin.

I stayed at work until noon, leaving a note on Thomas's desk stating that I was leaving for the day. I went straight to Wisconsin, alone.

I guess I wanted to shut this thing down on my own. I knew the last year had given everyone their share of emotional roller-coaster rides, and I thought that bringing anyone close to me might keep them on this ride longer than was necessary. The one ride I wanted was closure, at least from this part of it. I was still far away from the recovery I was hoping for, but I had enough sense to know that in order to somehow justify what he had done to me, I was sure Smith had described me as the devil from Chicago. I was sure he assumed I would arrive with a busload of friends and family from the Windy City. I remember thinking between the time I woke up that day and the time I left for Wisconsin that I wanted to prove Mr. Smith wrong, but I also looked at going alone as another step toward recovery.

No one had expected me when I arrived an hour before the 2:30 start. The district attorney was glad I came and assigned two deputies to me. He asked if I wanted to speak once we were in the hearing. I said, "I'll think about it." We went into the same courtroom in which the trial had taken place. On one side was Smith, his wife, kids, mother, father, twenty close friends, and, of course, his born-again minister. On my side were the district attorney, two deputies, and newspaper reporters. I just sat there, staring out the window at the bare Wisconsin trees, thinking it must be a bad movie or the worst dream possible. I was called upon by the judge to speak to Smith, so I did. I was not even the least bit nervous. This was the one time the brain injury actually came in handy.

One thing that I was aware of from the brain injury was that my sentences did not always come out of my mouth in the same order my brain had intended. By that I mean there were times when the right words came out in the wrong order, or I knew what I wanted to say, but the ability to speak those words correctly became extremely difficult. This is common in survivors with moderate to severe brain injuries. It is called Broca's aphasia, or motor aphasia. It was just one of those things I dealt with, and the only way for a Chicago native to deal with it was to talk very slowly. That being the case, I was more concerned with making sure the sentences came out right than I was about the crowd around Smith; it was somewhat surreal.

I spoke slowly, trying to make sure I thought through what I was saying. I knew that the slower I spoke, the better my chances were of having the words come out of my mouth in the order they were supposed to. I turned towards Smith and said, "I hope you realize what happened was a mistake that we will both have to live with. I don't know what will happen to you because of this. I am more concerned with getting back to the person I used to be; however, almost a year ago the doctors would have told you I would never have the ability to sit here and tell you what I am telling you, let alone drive here, so I am pleased with that progress. I know I still have a way to go." I paused, then continued on, "I do know that if you are punished, whatever sentence you're given is temporary; mine is permanent, but again, I have come a long way in the past year and plan to continue to get better. I hold no animosity and hope your life changes—mine sure did." My last statement was a quick story. I told them how I took my seven-year-old son, Jimmy, bowling a few weeks ago, and out of nowhere, Jimmy said, "I'm glad you didn't die, Dad, 'cause I'd have no one to play with."

With that I sat down, and I'm sure I had a complete look of relief on my face. I remember that feeling of relief like it was yesterday; but more than that, I was oblivious to the impact my statement had on the people in the courtroom.

No one on Smith's side would look at me, not even

the two morons from the trial who verbally harassed Mary Beth and me. The newspaper reporter was crying; the deputy leaned over to me and said, "That was the most powerful impact statement I have ever heard at a sentencing." The judge started yelling at Smith, and at the same time he stood up, crying, and said, "I never meant to hurt you. I made a mistake." I was just sitting there, emotionless for the first time in a year, but still puzzled at how dramatically different my life had become.

I was the first one out of the courtroom, accompanied by two police officers. I was told by the prosecuting attorney that the police officers would walk me to my car and give me an escort to the interstate. "No way," I said. "That's not necessary." They insisted. On the way to the car, the three of us were walking behind the building, and as we came to the end of the building, Smith's younger brother appeared out of nowhere. We all stopped. He stared at me. I stared back. Not in a mean or vindictive way, but in a way where we both said what we had to say without saying a word.

The police escorted me to the interstate and then waved off. I pulled over, plugged in the five-pound car phone UPS had given me in case I ever got lost, and called Mary Beth as I passed the sign that said, *Welcome to Illinois*. I didn't say much, just told her, "It's over. See you soon."

Nick Smith was sentenced to one year in prison. Although it felt like a weight had been lifted off me, it did not create closure for anything. I still had a lot of learning and adjusting ahead of me. I honestly had no idea how much adjusting I was going to have to do in an effort to get used to this new, somewhat modified version of me.

Now that the sentencing was behind me, I was hoping it was time to start over. I figured I would get better much quicker now that I had reached the one-year mark since the accident. As the following years would prove, that prediction was not even close.

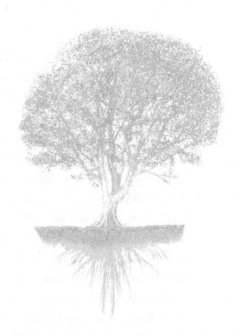

starting over

Starting over meant dealing with what the future had in store in for me. Most of what was in store was a mystery. One of the first steps in continuing my recovery was keeping in contact with my therapist from the rehabilitation school. I had become dependent on the facility and the therapist who had cared for me. To me, the school was like what a personal sponsor is to a recovering alcoholic.

I realize now when I look back that what I struggled with initially and still struggle with today is referred to as "executive functions." These are functions such as planning, organizing, abstract reasoning, problem solving, and making judgments. Recovery from cognitive deficits is greatest within the first six months after an injury and more gradual after that. I will always have problems or difficulties in those areas. Sometimes I experience these symptoms to a greater degree than at other times. I believe it depends on the amount of information I am trying to manage or comprehend as well as the amount of stress I am under. It can also be due to small factors, like how much rest I have had. An injured brain has to work harder to perform the same tasks as it had performed pre-injury, so getting proper rest is important.

Not long after 1993 ended, I was asked to attend a focus meeting at the rehabilitation facility where I had been a patient. This meeting was for former patients of the rehabilitation facility and their families. I was in for a big surprise. Obviously, the objective of the meeting was to talk about progress and share insight about your life.

After we all introduced ourselves to the group, I realized I was the only one there without a family member; more importantly, I realized why I was the only one without a family member. That reason was not that no one in my family would have attended; they would have had I asked. The reason was I was the only TBI survivor at that meeting who could drive. This was a real awakening. I felt blessed, yet at the same time I felt confused. Confused as to why I was the only one who was able to drive, and guilty.

The other patients began to talk about what their

life was like prior to their brain injury: "I was a dentist," said one; "I was a teacher," said another. They went on to describe what they did now in regards to employment or staying busy. For example, someone in the group went from being a six-figure professional to working part-time at a fast-food restaurant, and that was a big step for him. They were so proud. I tried too hard to make a difference in that meeting. I just wanted to make them feel like we were all the same, although I knew I was different due to some of the things I could still do. I left there thinking, *Maybe I am worse than I thought. Maybe I should not have the job I have, and maybe I should not be driving.* Someone at the meeting brought up that when one spouse suffers a brain injury, the marriage has an eighty percent chance of ending in divorce. *How come I am still married? Is she stuck with me? What did that trip to Wisconsin really do to me?* I had a perfect life before that trip, absolutely perfect... Well, I wished I were taller, but outside of that it was perfect.

After my accident, Mary Beth would always coach me in public. If we were out among friends or relatives, she would monitor what I said as well as try to prompt me to stop speaking. She did this because I would ramble on and on without reaching my point, or I would forget what I was talking about and just keep talking, sometimes about nothing. Early on, she would finish my sentences; then she would elbow me or just give me a look. I hated this, but it was part of relearning to adjust socially. My brain needed a remote control, and the problem was I did not have the ability to work the remote. I needed an autopilot.

Life was so unpredictable for me. One day I would recognize that I could do something better than I could the day before, and the next I would realize that I was still miles away from who I once was. Most bizarre was that the moods seemed to change faster, and the shift in emotions became an everyday occurrence. The adrenaline rushes I had were euphoric. It was as if this volcano of happiness would run through my veins. Unbelievable would describe it best. You could tell me my car was on fire, and I am sure I would have just laughed it off and moved on. I do have to admit that I occasionally looked forward to my brain going through this happiness emotion. Then there was the crash of that particular emotion, like someone just pulled the plug. I was also starting to get used to some of my coping mechanisms. For example, I carried very little with me. I would carry only one key, which would be for the car I was driving. I would never carry a wallet. Everything I did at work or at home always had to be placed in the same location. At UPS, everything I worked on went into a binder, and the binder went in the same place. At home, everything had to be positioned in the same spot; otherwise, I would never remember where anything was. I would write down on paper where I put things, and the paper would stay "on my dresser" or "in my car." I left myself notes everywhere. Remembering became a job, and it still is.

I began to realize that certain memories were gone. I know you can't remember everything; however, it became obvious after a while that certain events were erased. They could have happened the year before or three years ago; it didn't matter, because they were gone. My short-term memory was getting better but was nowhere near what it once was. Here is how it works: tell me your name, and maybe I will remember it. My best chance of remembering a name is to link it to something else. If you said your name was John, I would have a better chance of recalling it because I would remember that you have the same name as my brother. Tell me one thing, and there is a chance I can remember it based on the mood of my brain. Tell me two things and it gets a little fuzzy. Tell me three things to remember, and everything you've told me is flushed away. That is as prevalent today as it was then.

One particular coping method I used to keep my mind "excited" was trying to plan something that I would look forward to for months in advance. Patience was something that was lost and replaced with a strange version of obsessive-compulsive disorder. In other words, if I said I was going to do something, I did it, which I am not sure is always true with TBI survivors. One thing that was extremely hard, and is still today, was the ability to stay focused. It was an absolute fight to stay on one task or focus on one topic. I would have to say that it is still very difficult for me. What is more frustrating is staying focused during a conversation. While I am being told one thing, my brain is telling me something totally different. I just have such a short retention span and only recall a small portion of what you are saying that my brain *switches channels* and I'm gone. I could be, for example, listening to you talk and then walk away while you are in the middle of what you are saying. These difficulties are going to be with me for life. I just need to continue to find coping mechanisms.

I began to put things in front of me that were not material in nature, just things I was looking forward to, like having friends over for a 70's-themed party or landscaping the yard. Whatever it was didn't really matter; I just needed to keep my mind reminded of something I looked forward to. I truly believe this was a coping method for depression.

Here comes the future of living with a TBI. Yes, there were moments where, as long as I said very little, I seemed like the old me. It is amazing how good I became at learning how to hide deficits. You continue to recognize problems, and in my case, I became very good at acting. I realized that the next few years were going to be spent trying to convince people that there was nothing wrong with me; you really get quite convinced that the key to your future is being considered as normal. Again, the more you try to be normal, the more you realize that is not the case; however, I wasn't going to tell anyone.

As far as work, I was going with the flow and trying to learn how to find the shortest path to whatever it was I had to do without letting anyone realize that I struggled, and I struggled a lot. The therapist had warned me that I would wrestle with some of my deficits for life. One thing the therapist did around this time was to observe how I set up my work life. Again, the only way they thought I would be able to manage my life was to stay as simple and organized as I could. I could see organization was going to be a problem for me. I ended up putting everything I did in binders with huge letters on the side to help me identify the contents. This really laid the foundation for what I was going to have to learn to live with for the rest of my life. I remember thanking God that I was not driving a UPS package car like I did when I started. There was no way I could have done that job again, unless I had a route with one delivery, and that was not very likely.

Work was beginning to consist of sticking with what I could do best and figuring out ways to hide assignments that required skills I felt I didn't have anymore. The nice part of my job was I never had to use computers; we were still a few years away from that, but it was coming. I relied on friends at work who I knew were really good at things that I was not, or could provide information that would make my job appear a bit more fitting.

My manager, Thomas, who was outstanding with me, had been transferred and replaced by a gentleman named Shawn O'Leary. Shawn was a complete people-person and a natural-born leader. We used to say how we would run through a wall for that guy. Shawn was literally the ideal manager to work for, especially in regards to my continued recovery. Shawn always tried to utilize the positive skills each individual had, and his motivational abilities were always present. He was perfect for this time in my recovery. Shawn appreciated me for what I could do well, such as sales and client service, and understood that I struggled with some executive functions. He seemed to have a sense of how important any personal positive recognition was to me. That being the case, Shawn would always make sure he acknowledged my gains; however, he also recognized and provided me help with my weaknesses. Positive recognition for even the smallest task done well is worth a million dollars to a TBI survivor, especially in the early stages of recovery. One thing about Shawn was that he realized how important effort was and didn't always wait for a perfect result before giving someone a "pat on the back." He was that way with everyone, and we all appreciated it.

My emotions were becoming a little more reasonable. Yes, it was hard trying to figure out which emotion was going to show up in the next five minutes, but having the least amount of stress in your life is absolutely pivotal to some sort of normalcy for a TBI survivor.

One thing that soon becomes obvious during recovery is the need for organization, like my putting everything in the same place. That became the routine at work and at home. What you try to eliminate is the frustration that comes from not remembering. In my case, if I lost something or could not find it, I would become obsessed with finding that particular item, and the obsessive part was definitely not helpful. I began doing certain tasks on the same day of the week. Whether it was cutting the grass, washing the car, or work-related tasks, it did not matter. Repetition was important in obtaining some form of normalcy.

Since I always paid the household bills, I wanted to resume that activity. When I did, I needed to figure out a way to make sure I was up-to-date with my payments. I never really knew the best way, so I would keep experimenting until I figured out what worked, which was a filing system that had thirty-one files. When I received a bill, I would place it in a file that was seven days away from the due date. Each day I would check to see what was due, and it was always a relief to find an empty file.

I began to get accustomed to constant emotional changes; however, the up-and-down brain activity was hard to adjust to. I have always called it what it felt like, and it felt like my brain was on a roller coaster. I touched on this earlier; it is something that you get used to, but never completely. I believe the clinical phrase is *circular thinking*. This basically means your brain does not have the ability to filter what thoughts come in or how long you can hold onto a thought. It is also referred to as "a brain that is working too fast."

For years I have been told by others, "I wish I had your energy." What appears to be energy is really a lack of control. In my case, if a thought enters my brain, I have to go right to it. If I am mowing the lawn, and the thought flies through to wash the car and change the oil, I become obsessed with washing the car and changing the oil. What happens too often is that my brain wants to do too much; it generates a never-ending list of *to-do* items. I write the items down and check them off as they are completed. The mental benefit is that I remove them from my brain before becoming obsessed with getting the tasks accomplished.

My neighbor always comments on the fact that I

run everywhere. If I need something across the street or a block away, I run. The reason is that I finish what I need to get done in a shorter time span. Again, the more information I remove from the brain, the better. I just wish it would stop coming up with things to do. One of the downfalls to circular thinking is trying to sit still. It becomes extremely difficult to relax when your brain is running too fast. Imagine this coupled with obsessive-compulsion.

Depression was also difficult to deal with. It could hit me like a baseball bat. Too many nights I found myself sitting on the couch at four in the morning, wondering, *How I am going to get through this?* The depression would sometimes last a little longer than I could handle; I simply had no choice but to deal with it. At times like that I would try to come up with something that might temporarily remove the depression. Nobody has the same coping methods, and mine may seem odd at times, but they are mine and they worked for me. What I needed to do was become obsessed with something that would occupy my mind on the positive side, something that would help me escape whatever it was that was pulling me down. This became something I do to this day: find an escape. As much as I struggle staying focused, I have found that having something in the future that I look forward to is a form of personal medication.

One day a question came from Mary Beth that should have given me something to look forward to: "Do you want to have another baby?"

Mary Beth said that my recovery from the point I had

almost died had progressed to where there was enough of the old me showing up for her to believe that we could make it, and having another child seemed like something we should consider. I don't remember putting any more thought into it than saying "okay." Most things didn't shock me, and most often I seemed to be the one who provided the shocks. The doctors had told her during my recovery that having more children was not recommended. The reason the doctors had recommended that we avoid having another child was simple: they were almost certain that I would not be able to handle it. In most cases of damage to the left front temporal lobe, which controls your emotions among other aspects of your personality, there are concerns regarding your ability to deal with the stress of a newborn. So in the best interest of TBI survivors and their families, doctors strongly suggest giving the question of a new baby serious consideration, which we did.

After months of anticipation, on March 4, 1995, my son Brian was born. I cried the minute he came into my life. I viewed this as a major step in my search for peace in my new life. We brought Brian home, and he brought nothing but smiles to all of us. There was something about Brian that reminded me of myself. Mary Beth and I wanted another child, and we were very fortunate to be blessed with such a beautiful boy.

Looking back, I think all of us in my family needed Brian to bring some form of "newness" to our lives. I know I was still recovering, and so were they. This new life seemed to move us to the next step. It made it easier for me having the other kids, Katie and Jim, around to help out. Taking care of little Brian was pure fun; the kid was a breeze.

Things in my life now seemed to be somewhat manageable. My position at work consisted of working with some of our larger clients in an effort to grow the business while at the same time make sure we retained what business we had. The biggest thrill I received from working with my clients was converting them over to UPS. They sometimes would use us for some services and our competitors for others. I knew all my clients before the accident, so I think they saw the changes and always gave me a little slack when it came to dealing with their needs. As late as 1996, I didn't use computers at work, so I was mainly applying the skills I still had and making sure those abilities were focused on positively affecting my performance. That was also the year UPS began recognizing individual sales accomplishments with their Million Dollar Club sales awards. I was one of the first to receive the award. It was a great feeling to know that I was successful in my job despite my deficits.

There were quite a few positives since my TBI. My home life was busy, but I have to say it was very good and I felt like I understood my injury more with every year that passed. Mary Beth had made sure we survived through those first few years. I thought a lot about two managers I had worked for in the years immediately following my injury: Thomas Farrell in 1993, and then Shawn O'Leary through 1996. Until now, I never fully appreciated how understanding and insightful they were in managing and working with me. They both provided me opportunities to succeed, as well as room for me to continue to recover to the best of my ability. I was constantly learning to cope with my deficits as well as the reality of living with a TBI.

In regards to the sales and management positions I held at UPS, I felt I was successful in both of them. Shawn's understanding of what I faced, as well as his belief that a positive and supportive work environment was critical, helped me make tremendous strides. A little understanding coupled with positive reinforcement definitely made a difference in my ability to cope with, and in some cases reduce, the affects of my deficits. I was making a difference at work, and my home life was as close to normal as I could hope. The feeling I had knowing that I made a difference was priceless. Of course, as this injury has taught me, you never know what you have until it's gone.

There were two significant changes headed my way in 1996. In January, Shawn, my manager at UPS who helped me along in my recovery, was transferred. Shawn would be replaced with someone who was the complete opposite. His replacement's name was George, and he did not bear even a mild resemblance to Shawn. He seemed quite intense. However, I had always got along with everyone I worked for at UPS, so I was not really worried about it.

Shock number two: I guess someone upstairs thought that since we were doing so well with little Brian, we should have another baby. The new addition to the family was going to put all of us through some changes. We sold the home we were living in and moved to a bigger house. Both the new manager, George, and our new addition to the family were going to put my rehabilitating brain to the test, big time.

When 1996 began, I was still doing the same job I had for the past four years and was quite comfortable with my position. It also marked the beginning of year four in regards to my recovery. Change was difficult for me at times, especially at work. Not only was Shawn being transferred, but my position would be changing. For the most part, I would still be in sales; however, part of my position now included selling our services to potential clients who hadn't previously used our products. This may sound easy enough, but the clients I would be chasing were accounts others hadn't been able to win, due mostly to pricing by competitors that we would not even consider matching. I did appreciate the challenge. What would be a bit more difficult was the test my brain was going to go through. I had become comfortable with the people at the accounts I managed the past few years; they knew me, and I knew them. They knew I was not exactly who I used to be, but they accepted my shortfalls and knew I was determined to keep them satisfied. It would be a challenge leaving my comfort zone. The new target accounts would test my abilities.

With my deficits, retaining new information was challenging, and names were very hard to remember; I was still using the "buddy" reference for those whose names escaped me. My emotions were still out of line at times, and I could experience all of them in a small amount of time, but my temper was getting much better. One thing I had to constantly deal with was migraine headaches. I always had a pretty good idea when one was on its way. My face would start to sweat, dark circles would form under my eyes, and I would zone out as the pain increased. Usually I would make it home, and if I could not I just pulled over and lay in the car, popping as many aspirins as possible.

When I made it home, my family knew exactly what to do: make sure the bedroom was dark and there was a fan in the room. Have a cold wet rag for my face, and bring me something cold to drink. I would also have to prop plenty of pillows underneath my legs. The reason for this goes back to the hospital. When I was in intensive care, they elevated my legs. This continued to be the case when I returned home, and to this day I cannot sleep unless my legs are elevated.

Nineteen ninety-six started out with adjusting to a change in my job description as well as to a new department head. He certainly was not going to win any people skills awards. I continued to marvel at what happened to me while trying to figure out ways to outsmart my deficits. You never stop thinking about this type of injury because you are reminded of its existence every day, either through medication or doing something that doesn't seem quite right. There were days I felt really good: times when things seemed to be heading in the right direction.

My father and I had a peculiar bond. Nine months

before my brain injury, my father suffered a severe stroke. A few weeks prior to my injury, my brothers and I sat down with him in an effort to get him to continue therapy. I remember seeing him in the hospital, where I would also become a patient, and I was floored at the effect the stroke had on him. He couldn't speak, he was paralyzed on one side, and he always appeared confused. As he recovered, his speech came back and the paralysis faded, but he was not the same. He went from lively and talkative to quiet and very reserved. He didn't appear to know what was going on around him. However, after my ordeal I grew to understand what he was going through, and nothing he did or said ever struck me as strange.

Weeks after my brothers and I spoke with him, there I was, in the intensive care unit of the same hospital, with a severe brain injury. Certainly not something my dad and I wanted to have in common.

Before my injury, I remember my family being confused by my dad's actions. But after my injury, a year or so later, I felt like I understood him so well. I guess I knew what others in my family would hopefully never know: what it's like to live after a brain injury or stroke. I really, truly viewed him differently, and I felt sorry for my dad. I could see that he struggled with the realization that his life was different and he was no longer who he once was. Nonetheless, I was sure glad I had him around. He was never able to adjust to what happened to me; he seemed to block it out. He did get a bit better every year, and in 1996 we saw some signs of the "old Dude."

My new manager, George, was just getting settled

into his new position, so I really didn't have that much interaction with him. However, he did ask me, since I was a Chicago native, to drive him to some areas he was considering moving to. I gladly granted that request. While we were out looking at neighborhoods, we stopped by my house, and I introduced him to Mary Beth. He actually seemed nice and had begun to speak with Mary Beth as I exited the kitchen. During this conversation, all of his questions were focused on my brain injury. He wanted to know everything that was different about me in comparison to the pre-injury version. I was out of the room so I had no idea that this was happening. When I returned to the kitchen, George and I left.

When I returned home that evening, Mary Beth met me at the door and she had a worried look on her face. She began telling me about the conversation she had with George and how troubled she was about his questioning. I remember her saying, "This is not going to be good for you."

I really did not have many encounters with George until a meeting he held with all the managers, of which I was one. He asked me, for no reason, to name everything I had done at work the prior week. I told him that it was impossible for me to do so without my planner, but he just kept at it. I knew my fellow managers felt as uncomfortable with his interrogation as I did. I just couldn't answer any of his questions.

After the meeting, I requested a one-on-one conference with him. I explained in detail the reasons for my inability to provide him with all the answers he demanded. I tried to structure my words in a way so that he understood that I could do the job; I just couldn't do certain things as well as before my TBI. I asked him never to embarrass me again with similar questioning.

I had heard stories that were being circulated at work regarding some not-so-pleasant encounters he was having with my co-workers; however, this was my first work- related confrontation with him. In a strange way, the fact that I had heard others comment on his negative demeanor felt somewhat comforting. It just so happened that my brain injury was his weapon of choice when it came to me, and it was just the beginning. I decided it was in my best interest to start keeping notes of our conversations.

I recall that during one meeting when George was doing his usual "beat you into submission" ritual, which he was extremely good at, I stopped him. I had a faint burst of confidence and said right to his face, "I have spent the last three years trying to somehow rebuild my life and at the same time regain some form of confidence, and I will not let you take that away from me."

I know anger had something to do with that burst of confidence, but sometimes you surprise yourself. I never regretted saying that. Although it got me nowhere with George, it did get me somewhere in my mind. He didn't say much after that and neither did I, and that is all I care to remember about that first meeting.

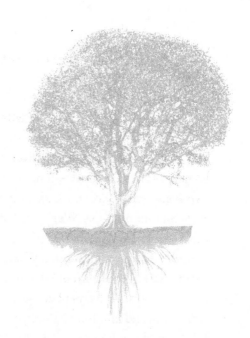

a life-changing addition

In December 1996, little Jennifer was born. She was a blonde-haired blue-eyed peanut. I would like to say that everything about her was perfect, and it's true…the one exception being that she preferred to cry between the hours of two and six in the morning. We sold the house in Tinley Park and bought one in an adjacent town called Mokena, one of the smaller suburbs outside of Chicago.

We found a nice place to build, and our home would be ready by the spring of 1997.

Another Christmas came, and like every one before, we celebrated it in my mom and dad's home on Christmas Eve. This was the happiest day of my dad's year, every year. My two brothers, who lived out of town, would come in for the holiday—John from Missouri with his two daughters, Lori and Lisa, and Steve and his family from Southern Illinois. We showed off little Jennifer while my dad wrapped my mom's gift in his workroom, just as he did every year. John usually helped my dad wrap my mom's portable vacuum or whatever he had picked up at Ace Hardware. I always made sure to walk into my dad's workroom and film John helping him prepare Mom's gift. John would laugh non-stop during the wrapping process. It was always fun to see everyone together. One thing was different: my dad seemed tired. He was mentally the best we had seen him since his stroke a few years earlier, but was tired.

January came, and again my brothers would come back into Chicago for a friend's Super Bowl party. I think this was my dad's second favorite day of the year. The Super Bowl, as we all know, was held on a Sunday, and my brothers would arrive on Saturday.

On this particular Saturday morning, I was with my son Jim at a baseball clinic. After it was finished, I was going to take Dad to see my new house that was under construction. The frame was up and we could walk around in it, and I knew he would be proud.

When I arrived home from the baseball clinic, Mary

Beth's car was in the driveway. This was very strange because she was supposed to be at work. It was 1997, and we did not have cell phones. As Jim and I walked into the house, Mary Beth met me in the kitchen. She had tears in her eyes, so I knew something was wrong. She informed me that my dad had passed away that morning. He had died in his sleep.

I guess his death was a test for me. I know I drove him crazy when I was a teen, as most teenagers do their parents. My grades were not where they could have been, my hair was too long, some of the beverages my friends and I drank were intended for individuals over twenty-one, and he was not happy that I didn't go to college. My three brothers had graduated from college, and he fully expected me to go. However, we became best friends after I got married.

I know he was proud of my family and my success at UPS. We did as much as we could together the last ten years of his life, and it was a great decade of memories for me. When I remodeled someone's house, he was there. We bowled in the same league. Every time my son Jim had a game, Dad was there. I remember Jimmy telling me how hard it would be to look in the stands and not see Grandpa. The fact that we did all these things together, coupled with the struggles of having a stroke that only I could relate to, made his passing easier on me. I told him as often as I could how much I loved him, especially after his stroke. I had no regrets, and I knew he was at peace.

That year went by quite fast. I moved the family to Mokena, Illinois, which was only seven miles from our previous address, but as far as the kids were concerned, it may as well have been seventy miles. They had to go to new schools, meet new friends, and Jim had to join a completely different baseball league. My focus was going to be on keeping my eleven-year-old boy happy. I put him in guitar school right away. I figured it would keep his mind off the move, at least for a half hour. I would drive him to guitar lessons and wait for him in the car. Most of the time I was able to stay put without going crazy. I would take this time to think. I mostly thought about the past few years and how different life had become in such a short amount of time.

I eventually and largely subconsciously began to adapt to some of my deficits and was starting to make my adjustments a way of life. There still were things I was never going to get used to—ever. Right after my accident, or at least the first few years, nobody in my family wanted to talk about it with me. Mary Beth would always tear up; my mom still says it was the worst thing she has ever gone through. Steve still gets mad when the topic comes up. Mike and John began to shed some light on some of the things I had said and done. Mike also began to tell me what the doctors had told him about my prognosis. As far as the friends who were there when I was injured, only Kevin would talk about it. He always had this one line every time I would get upset; he would tap my head with his hand and say, "Watch the head." Only he could do it and get a laugh out of everyone, including me.

Work was going okay, and I was doing everything I could to be successful at my position. George was busy making other people's lives miserable, and he had not targeted me yet. One day in July of 1997, while I was attending a two-day work meeting, I began to write about the past few years. I wrote as though someone across from me had just asked me how my brain injury occurred. I started writing on the first day of this meeting and didn't stop for ten years. I wrote about how the fateful trip began and I just kept going. It felt so good to write about it that I never wanted to stop. I went through my medical records, the court records, the get-well cards—you name it, I used it all as reference material. The cards Jimmy and Katie wrote still create a liquid-like substance in my eyes. I have every newspaper article written about my injury, including the original paper I used when I began writing this story. When I wrote, it felt like I was telling someone what my life was like, good and not so good, and it felt like I was being understood. Writing became an activity I used as a coping mechanism. To this day, when I am stressed, I write.

I became obsessed with this story, and every chance I got I sat down and rewrote it, and I didn't care if anyone ever read it. I realized that it was amazing to me because of what people told me about what happened. Ninety-nine percent of those around me will never know what I struggle with. If something about me does not seem right it is most often referred to as a *personality issue*. I believe I wanted to relive through conversation what had happened to me: *What did I look like? What did I say? When I had seizures, what would my body do? What would I say when you were able to wake me? Did I make you cry? If so, why did I make you cry?* I wanted to know everything. I wanted to see me as I went through this ordeal. I just wished I could watch a video of it all. Where was a show called "America's Most Puzzling Home Videos" when I needed it?

I began talking about the whole life experience with anyone who would listen, which, in hindsight, I realize may have been a mistake. I was so amazed with it all. My original therapist and doctors have told me that I am at the extreme when it comes to talking about my brain injury. Most TBI survivors never want to talk about it, or would not know how to talk about it. I wanted to help others who had brain injuries; maybe I could be a ray of hope. I was quite proud of what I had written and wanted everyone to read it. The problem was not everyone wanted to, at least not family members or friends. I didn't know why then, but I understand now. I wanted to remember what they wanted to forget.

I went back to the trauma center in Chicago, which was the third hospital I was in after the injury, because I wanted to see where I once was. I knew which floor I was on, the fourth, so I made my way up. I wanted to see what people with recent injuries looked like, how many machines they were hooked up to, and what their family's facial expressions were communicating. I don't know why this was so important to me; I believe it was a rediscovering of my life. I wanted to know what I went through. I would never wish this upon anyone, so I will never understand why I wanted to see what others looked like after their accidents. I feel bad about that, but it was a time in my life that just had to happen.

A nurse approached me in the hallway as I was sticking my head into the rooms, trying to make it look like I was looking for someone. I remembered the floor due to my dad's stroke, since he was also an alumnus of the same hospital. She asked if there was something she could help me with.

I explained that I was a once a patient here and wanted to meet someone who may have worked there at the time I was hospitalized. I wanted to see where I once was. She said that she had worked there at the time, but she needed more to go by. I told her that when I was awake I would ring the nurse bell and scream, "Get me a cab!" I reminded her that I was supposed to have brain surgery, but I took a turn for the better an hour or so before. Just as she began to put her hand over her mouth, another nurse walked up. She took her hand away from her mouth and said, "I remember you, I remember you." She told the other nurse who I was, and she remembered me as well. They said I was one of the patients whose stay they could not forget. I imagine my family had something to do with that. They were shocked that it was me. "We had you written off," one of them replied.

After we finished talking, they walked me down to the intensive care unit. One of them pointed to a bed and said, "That is where you were." I asked when they had removed the TV that was above the bed. They laughed and said that there never was a TV above the bed. For some reason, I remember a TV on a wall. Maybe it was a heat monitor…who knows? The experience felt like walking down memory lane; the only problem was, I didn't remember it. I began to feel like I had a multiple-month blackout.

At UPS, a job change was coming. I was going to be assigned as an Area Sales Manager. This was not a promotion but a lateral move. My manager George had told me that it would be a good match because I might be tired of what I was doing, and my experience in sales made it a natural fit. I went home and told Mary Beth about the change, which I was quite happy with, although I was not sure I had the ability to keep track of myself, let alone eight others.

I am sure you have heard the phrase *rain on your parade;* I believe the next sentence qualifies. The day after telling me I was a "good fit" for the new job, George had called me into his office to discuss an issue he had regarding my previous position. He was not happy with one area of my performance. I'm not sure why he waited until the day after he assigned me my new position to tell me this. After he was finished voicing his discontent, George told me he would let me know Christmas morning, which was five weeks away, if I would still be an employee at UPS.

I believed I had the capacity to do the job. There might be some areas I found challenging, but I was sure that I could handle the position. Initially I was somewhat worried that managing other people would be a problem because of my deficits. I had managed groups of sales representatives prior to my injury, but had been responsible only for myself since the injury. The good side was, I would be managing experienced account executives. They were using laptop computers, which I still had no idea how to use. I put the skills I had to use. I knew they were intimidated by George, so I said, "Forget about him. Let's just try to have some fun with the job."

I became the project person. Even though I was their manager, I hated the title and did not like being referred to as their boss, not my style. The first thing I did was put together a night out; we were going to spend Friday night at an indoor paintball arena. I thought a night out together would be a good team-building exercise. We had a great time and as far as I was concerned, we were off to a good start.

The following Monday I asked each person in my segment to provide me a list of what he or she felt was needed in order to increase our chances of being successful. The list ranged from new printers to placing a lock on the office where we would meet at the end of the day. I was fortunate enough to get approved the majority of what they requested. I was enjoying this position, and the fact that they all were very experienced made managing the segment somewhat easier. My job, as I saw it, was to report all the good things my account executives had accomplished and to provide assistance where and when I could. I was not interested in criticizing what could have been done better, but practiced constant positive recognition. Christmas came around, and my manager George never called, which meant he let me keep my job. I guess it was the season.

The good thing about being at a company for so long

was that I began to realize who I could turn to when I needed help or had problems. The job of selling or managing sales was getting more complicated as our portfolio of services and technology solutions expanded. It was a challenge for me digesting everything. As I said earlier, you really use the best of what you have and hide what skills or cognitive abilities you struggle with.

One aspect of brain injuries that I find incredibly strange is the effect on emotions. I know I have mentioned the impact the injury had on my emotions; however, the way it affects your emotions is what interests me. What I find remarkable, and, I might add, this is very "normal" for brain injury survivors, is that the injury amplifies your emotions. Although my brain was permanently damaged, there are areas that have become what they once were and more. For example, I have covered the anger, or rage as some have referred to it; however, there is also the complete opposite response. If pre-injury a situation or event that would have naturally caused me to get excited, post-injury I become euphoric. It was like happiness gone wild. The mood was magical, unlike any you could imagine. If I could bottle it and sell it, my finances would never again be an issue.

Of course, there is a distant cousin of the emotion happiness, and that unwelcome relative is depression. It falls under the same scenario as the other emotions; pre-injury depression was hard on me. Post-injury depression is horrible. It can literally paralyze me, especially if stress is involved. Typically, when stress is also present, most of my skills disappear. It can trigger any of the unpleasant emotions, including rage. It took me years to develop effective coping skills for depression, and unfortunately they don't always work. It doesn't take much to cause it, and you never know when your brain is going to process thoughts or circumstances that will put you into a depressed state. I could be having a great day, my brain could be in complete euphoria, and out of nowhere, like sticking a pin in a balloon, the euphoria is gone. Hello, depression.

By 1998, I was getting pretty good at the "managing a brain injury" game. Of course, I realize now that having less to manage in life is the best medicine for a TBI survivor. Unfortunately, at that stage of the game I was nowhere near figuring this out. I was still trying to get involved in as much activity as I could, but a side effect of being active was that I would lose track of things I was doing; they simply disappeared from my mind's radar. That is why I made sure I wrote down what I needed to do or what I was planning to do. It really is helpful. I just needed to place the list in the same place every time I added or deleted something. The last thing I needed was the frustration of forgetting where I put my "to do" list.

One deficit I really needed to stay on top of was that I could lose track of any conversation I was involved in, especially if it went on too long. At first I would panic when this would happen, and early on I really did not have a strong coping mechanism. As I mentioned earlier, initially when Mary Beth was around, she would help me stay on track or nudge me when I made my point. The nudge was a nice way of telling me to close my mouth.

What happens, and sometimes I knew when it was going to happen, is that I can be having a conversation with someone, and I pause. When I pause, there is a risk that the topic of the conversation may disappear.

This deficit is still prevalent today, though my ability to develop coping mechanisms has lessened the impact. It still can be frustrating, though not as much as it was initially. There were times where I would start a new conversation about a completely different topic. I suppose the individual I was talking to just let it go. Today I will say to whomever I am talking to, "I'm sorry, I don't remember what I was saying," or, "I lost my place." The best method for me is to try and shorten the time it takes me to complete my statement. If I do lose track I politely ask, "Could you please tell me where I left off, or what exactly were we talking about?"

This problem gave birth to another difficulty: making sure I don't talk out of turn when involved in conversation. If I was in a conversation with two or more people, and I was actually keeping track of a particular moment in the conversation and had something to add, I would blurt it right out. If I didn't blurt it out, I knew I would forget what it was I wanted to say, and maybe, just maybe, I would have something to add. It would drive me nuts to know that I was going to do it; I just had no defense for it. The sad part is I still don't, but I am somewhat more tactful now with this deficit. It really is hard to control because I want to be sure to say what I want to say before my brain moves the thought to the "storage bin."

I want to mention that up to this point as I have

highlighted some of my deficits from this injury you may think, *I do the same thing.* To some degree, I am sure that everyone does some of what I have discussed; I just do it all the time and, most likely a bit more severely.

I should emphasize here that I also do a lot of things very well. I am considered to be quite creative, have good people skills, and most think I have a good sense of humor—dry, but good. I am outstanding at sales, which is what I did before my injury, and I always truly enjoyed it. I have had to relearn what made me successful. I realized that experiencing any success from my efforts was extremely helpful in moving my progress along. I became surprisingly good at knowing where to get answers, but sometimes not very good at remembering or storing the information once I obtained it. I never bothered with trying to remember trivial or unimportant information, since my ability to retain new data was severely reduced due to the injury. I call this type of irrelevant information "brain clutter," and I do not like clutter. I have become selective in what I attempt to remember.

I became good at being whomever I needed to be based on the situation. I honestly believe that individuals I have met since my brain injury who never got to know me very well would give different descriptions about *whom* they met. I have given people impressions of me that most likely were not *me.* Most often, this would happen if I was experiencing euphoria. I would speak a thousand words a minute and at the same time have a burst of energy waiting to come out of my body. Or they could have met the "absolutely no patience" version, which typically makes its way to the angry, not-so-nice version. Then there is the version of me that seems to be quite normal, provided all areas of the brain, damaged and not damaged, are working as best as they can. When this happens, it is a great feeling, and I most often don't realize it is there until it leaves. It does not happen often enough.

What most often triggers the euphoric mood for me is the recognition of something I did well. As a lot of self-confidence is lost with specific types of brain injuries, situations where one is recognized for an accomplishment can spark euphoria. In my case, self-confidence eroded more the further I was from the injury date. The reason for this is simple: until the brain begins to recognize the differences pre-injury versus post-injury, a TBI survivor tends to believe all is well. However, when you begin to realize that you can no longer do some things as well as before, that you are a different person, or that people may think less of you, your self-confidence really takes a beating.

What helps me, well, or at least what I find relaxing, is being alone, whether I am building something, landscaping, or driving. I think about life, and I try to focus on ways to make life better. A major part of what helps me through situations is music that speaks to what I may be going through. I have always made music part of my life, and I have always associated it with important times in my life or the moods I may experience. Certain words in specific songs helped me get through tough times. I guess if it works, stick with it.

I chose not to take the prescription drugs that my

doctors recommended. They did not agree with my approach; however, by 1998 I was on year five of my recovery, and I thought I was doing okay. I was on several prescription drugs the first year of my injury, but my goal was not to take any medications. I believed that if I took drugs for my injury, I would not be beating it on my own. This is not something I would recommend, but every TBI survivor is different in his or her approach. I am not saying that mine was right, but being stubborn and assuming that I was winning, the doctors were not going to change my mind.

I am sure that others close to me saw a struggling or different version of me. The struggling version was much more apparent under stressful or unfavorable conditions. I have been told that it was hard to stress me out pre-injury; post-injury was a different story. More times than not, I was stressed; sometimes I hid it well, and sometimes I didn't. One of the causes of stress for me was that too many thoughts could go through my brain at the same time. Trying to sort out everything that I was thinking and maybe getting lucky enough to prioritize all those thoughts was borderline impossible. I could really lose it under stress, which is common among TBI survivors.

Being on year five of my recovery, I thought the worst years were behind me and the future was bright. As every year ended, I always believed the next year could only get better. I only had one direction to go, and that direction was going to be nothing but positive. Of course, if that was going to be the case, I could stop writing and give you a quick fairy-tale ending.

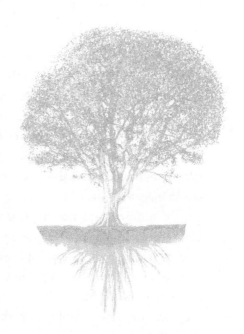

progress made,
progress lost

The year 1997 began a period where my recovery often seemed to move in reverse, and where a supportive work environment was replaced by one that was stressful and often hostile. On the positive side, my home life was busy and felt somewhat normal. There was plenty to do in the new house. I completed the finishing work on my basement, so that had kept me occupied. Physical work seemed to be quite rewarding for me. It kept my mind engaged in a good way, which I appreciated, as did everyone else. There really was minimal cognitive activity involved, so I never seemed to get fatigued as I did with activities where I needed to use the damaged areas of my brain. Working, on the other hand, would become interesting. I enjoyed the position of managing the sales executives for the national sales segment. However, Shawn, the manager whom I had been so successful under and greatly admired, was now in Atlanta. His replacement, George, would prove to be a totally different story.

I began to have a few unpleasant interactions with George again. Funny thing about this guy was, he was quite smart with the way he ran the department; it was the quest for power combined with some strange people skills that was his enemy—or our enemy. Some of our differences seemed to result from his attitude that I was an outsider when working with the other eight managers. George once told me, "They go this way; you purposely go the other way." He also said, "When I call you down to my office, you walk; they run." Hey, safety first. It was true, I did things my way, and I stuck with what worked for me, not anyone else. I always got along well with those I worked with; I just was not into "cliques" at work. I interacted well with my co-workers, but I was not a follower. Nobody knew my limitations better than I did. I worked with the tools that got me through the day.

One particular phrase came out of George's mouth more than I cared to hear. Before I tell you why he said it the first time, I will admit to some of the blame for not writing down what I needed to remember. As I have said, if you tell me one thing, I'm okay; more than one item, and I really have to be sure to mentally frame it or write it down. However, the problem that existed then, and to this day, was I got overconfident with my memory, and when this happens, I assume I can remember whatever I was told. If I repeat it all the way to my desk and immediately write it down, there is a good chance I will remember; however, if I encounter someone and a conversation takes place, that information disappears. Once in a great while it will come back to me days later, and along with that comes panic. I panic because often the time frame required to do what I was asked has passed.

The phrase that came out of George's mouth when I failed to remember one of his assignments was "You and that damn brain injury." As much as I thought it was a bit out of line, it didn't shock me at the time. When it became a catchphrase he used to address me, it became a problem.

The problem with these *damn brain injuries* is discussing your limitations or special considerations with those you work for. Based on my experience, it is sometimes viewed as presenting an excuse. In most situations, I was afraid of bringing up that there were areas I was struggling with due to my brain injury. I would get this feeling that certain managers would condescendingly refer to me in regards to my brain injury and look for ways to get me off the payroll.

After a few more encounters with George, which resulted in repeated "You and that damn brain injury" jabs, I made a visit to the Human Resources department.

I gave the Human Resources manager two pages of notes regarding our interactions. Upon reading my notes, the manager said, "You aren't going to sue us, are you?"

"No," I replied. "I just don't want to have my brain injury brought into our discussions any more, and I am asking you or someone on your level to review this with him." I also asked that he not hold my brain injury against me.

The information I provided the Human Resources manager was then reviewed with George. He called me into his office for a round-table meeting, not an across-the-desk meeting. George began by telling me what the Human Resources department told him. I listened as best I could as he apologized, and at one point he began crying. George admitted that he had no right to say those things, and he hoped that I accepted his apology, which I did at the time. Here is what that brief meeting actually meant: no more abuse for a while. That was what I sensed a week or two after the meeting, and I was quite sure I was going to be right.

I will admit that there were times I am sure I caused others to become frustrated with me. I was frustrated with myself quite often, but I kept going. What would frustrate me was trying to keep my mind focused while someone was talking to me or while I was trying to concentrate on a specific work task. Let me try to simplify this concept: my brain's memory or ability to retain new information went from a houseful of capacity to a closetful. There were times I would stare at whomever was speaking and just pray that something they said would stick in my mind.

I would get so stressed trying to remember that I would break down and forget everything. Now there were times when the conversation was short and I would be okay; however, by short I mean twenty or thirty seconds. So yes, I understood why George or anyone else would get frustrated with me if I had appeared to ignore something they had told me. Most often, I am sure it was assumed I just forgot out of convenience or stupidity. I can assure you this was not the case.

There was something else I struggled to understand: the better my group of sales executives performed, the more frustrated George became with me. My group was doing outstanding; we were all working as a team, and their career experience made my job quite manageable. As far as could tell I was doing okay with the managing side, so I was confused with his frustration.

I was discussing this with a fellow manager, who shed some light on this weird situation. His name was Brad and what he told me, very discreetly, was, "George put you in this position to fail. The national segment was not supposed to make its business plan and you were put in place to take the hit. George did not believe you had the ability to manage people." Brad was a good friend of mine and he told me this for my own benefit. I used that statement as motivation to succeed. For some reason it didn't bother me as much as it probably should have: I just chose to take it for what it was worth.

My segment kept working hard, but George and I were ready for a new battle. The comments regarding my brain injury, coupled with his disbelief that any shortfalls in my day-to-day activities were related to my injury, was something that had to stop. UPS was a tough place for anyone to work, let alone someone with a brain injury. By design, UPS has always given their management multiple tasks. UPS provides their employees excellent training so they are prepared to handle multiple responsibilities, and very rarely was there one primary function I was responsible for in my job. UPS prides itself on having a management force that can multitask better than any other in the industry. That being the case, it is tough for a TBI survivor, because multitasking is not something that you do well after a brain injury. Multiple moods or personalities are unfortunately common, but multitasking is definitely not on the list of "things I can still do well." The issue with multitasking is that I may have difficulty prioritizing the tasks that are given, and there are times when I may jump from one task to the next. The battle was at hand, and it was one for the record books.

The abuse or hostility from George gradually made its way back into my work life. Due to his frustration with me, coupled with his lack of belief in regards to my injury, I had to do something. I called Linda Muller at Cognitive Rehabilitation Specialists and discussed the situation with her. I always kept her up to date in regards to how my life was going, so she had an idea on what I should do. Linda suggested, and I agreed, that I could offer to submit to neurological testing to provide George proof of my disability. She would arrange the tests. I made this offer to George, and without hesitation he agreed.

I would have the test performed in October 1998 at

the University of Illinois Chicago Medical Center, and when the results of the tests were finalized we would meet with the District Human Resource manager. Linda also suggested that I meet with a board-certified neuropsychologist, and I agreed. A neuropsychologist is a psychologist who specializes in studying brain behavior relationships. At the University of Illinois, I was to meet with a doctor whom Linda referred to as an expert in the field of brain injuries. I have always been anxious prior to going into a doctor's office. I hoped that they would tell me my brain injury was mysteriously gone.

I would need a total of six days for the tests, three at the University of Illinois and three with the neuropsychologist. The neuropsychologist visits came first. As much as I was curious about the tests and the results, that I had to take them to prove I was disabled was ridiculous.

The tests proved interesting. I recall being blindfolded and placed in front of a board with geometric shapes cut out of it. The shapes were triangles, circles, squares, and so on. The pieces that were to go into these holes were put in front of me. I was instructed to place the pieces in the holes as fast as I could. Other tests included audio memory assessment. I was told a short story, and then I was asked several questions regarding the story. The point of this was to evaluate how much of the story I had retained. There was also a personality test. This test was not designed to determine if I actually had a personality; it was designed to assess various dimensions of my personality. I am sure they called it something other than a personality test. This and other testing went on for two days by associates of the neuropsychologist. After the test results were tabulated, I was to meet the doctor. I didn't see her until the day the results were to be reviewed, and it felt like I was meeting the *Wizard of Oz.*

The doctor had a lengthy conversation with me. She wanted to know what I did for a living, what I struggled with, what I did well, and so on. When I told her what I did for a living, she looked shocked. She told me she guessed I was an architect, which was odd, since I don't remember designing houses during the testing. We talked for a long time before she revealed the results of the tests that I had taken. We discussed my childhood, my relationship with my parents when I was a kid—you name it, we talked about it.

One thing she asked me was if I ever planned on going to college. I told her that I wished I had my degree in the event that I ever wanted to pursue a different career or change employers. She told me not to plan on attending college because I would never remember what was discussed in class. The doctor explained that going to college would cause additional frustration because the testing indicated that my ability to retain new information was severely damaged. She base her opinion on the tests as well as the medical records and her observation of me during our conversation. Not going to college didn't bother me as much as the reason why I should not. She told me that I had approximately ten percent of my original capacity to remember new information.

We talked about my memory problems, or what I thought were memory problems. She explained to me that my memory was satisfactory; it was my inability to recall new information that was severely impaired. Here is how it was worded in the written test results: "Memory for new verbal information is severely impaired, with retention of paragraph-length material at the first percentile on immediate recall and after a half-hour delay." The test went on to say, "He is easily overwhelmed if given more than very small amounts of information at any given time, though he does profit from repeated exposure to verbal material."

The test results continued to outline the need to have repeated exposure to new information in order to obtain any degree of retention. That somehow made sense to me and at the same time cleared up a lot of my perception of what was going on. The tests did say that I had an excellent visual memory, which was consistent with my experience. I actually did remember information such as phone numbers or addresses if they were written down or printed on paper rather than told to me. I always felt like I photographed the number in my mind. I really did not comprehend this until we talked about it. I was getting better at audio memory for simple things, such as names. The reason I was getting better, and I mentioned this earlier, was because I learned to link new information to something that was already familiar. It really helped me. I am not sure if it was the additional thinking involved in this process that helped my memory, or whether it was attributable to linking a new memory with an old one. Either way, it was working.

The tests showed that I was excellent at problem

solving, which may explain why my coping methods were very effective. I was always a good problem solver, and I tried not to look at my deficits as permanent impairments. I viewed them as temporary problems with potential solutions. It made no sense to believe that I would never be able to figure out a way to solve certain problems. Early on in my recovery, I believed my deficits were temporary problems. I knew that identifying all my deficits was impossible then, and it is impossible now. With time, I realized that permanent coping methods were going to be a part of life because my deficits would be with me for life. That reality becomes more comprehensible with time.

In regards to my memory issues, or *new information-retrieval* problems, the doctor provided me a list of ways to compensate for this deficit. She told me that my memory is not a muscle that can be exercised, and attempts at practicing to remember would not be helpful. Instead, here is what she suggested:

1. Take notes when possible. This is cumbersome because he cannot tell what he will store and what he will not, and it is not possible to write everything. However, making notes, perhaps on a laptop computer, about important things to remember or of things he plans to do would be helpful.

2. He might wish to try to learn speedwriting to take notes more efficiently.

3. He may want to tape record meetings with his boss and department for later reference.

4. When he attempts to master new verbal information (either auditory or written), he should keep learning sessions very brief and alternate them with other (even physical) activities.

5. He requires more than the usual amount of over-learning. Overlearning is repeated practice after initial mastery of the material. We all must do some overlearning to store new information, but he needs more than the usual.

6. Because he constantly has to compensate for these memory storage problems, he fatigues easily, and stress affects him more than it would the average individual.

7. What he describes as problems with attention are actually these memory storage problems. He feels he has difficulty attending when actually he is overloaded with new information.

The neuropsychologist went on to say that I had an outstanding recovery from my brain injury, and most of my abilities remained strong. She stated that the problems I had presented me with a very significant challenge. Included in her closing comments was the statement that she felt I was anxious to please others and willing to put forth whatever effort was required to do well on my job. She said I needed the approval of others (I think that was a nice way of saying I am insecure) and having the understanding of my supervisors of my very specific problems was important. Conversely, she felt that disapproval caused increased stress and tended to impede in my functioning.

Now I suppose I could have put all of that on a shirt or on a business card, but somehow I didn't think it would have helped. I wasn't quite sure what I was capable of after this assessment. Sure, I had some strong skills, but the biggest challenge I had was one nobody could see or understand. That was a problem. I used to say that if I had some form of physical deficit as a result of my injury, I might be better off.

Now that the cognitive testing was done, it was off to the University of Illinois for neuro-physical testing. This was something my initial therapist from rehabilitation always wanted me to do. When Linda Muller set it up, she talked about the doctor I was going to see, Dr. Gaviria, and how well versed he was with brain injuries and assessing deficits. Despite my anxiety, I was hoping they would tell me how much better I was. Again, I might as well hope for the best.

The test started out with the doctor's intern asking me pages of questions. You never know what the right answer is, and sometimes you think it's a game. There were also basic brain-assessment tests. They would try to gauge my ability to think, how fast I thought, how difficult it was for me to think, and at what level my brain performed. I always hoped I would find out something new about my brain's ability or more information about my deficits.

The afternoon test consisted of actual scans and tests of the brain. I was brought into a room for the first test, and it was obviously going to be a long one. I was strapped to a board so that my head would not move. Then dye was injected into my veins so that it would run through my brain. I was told to sleep or be still; just don't move. The purpose of the test was to see how easily the dye flowed through the veins in my brain, and it took quite some time. I was dying to know the results. You just hope there are no roadblocks or traffic jams in the brain.

The following day, Mary Beth and I went to the University of Illinois to review the tests with Dr. Gaviria. The test showed that I had blood flow problems on the left side of the brain and irregularities on the right side. Dr. Gaviria continued to review all his findings as well as a review of the verbal testing. His assistant was present and bobbed his head at everything the doctor said.

He told me one thing that was puzzling at first but made sense the more he explained it. Dr. Gaviria said that my brain runs too fast, and I should consider taking specific medicine designed to slow it down. I was not sure what he meant by *runs too fast,* so I asked him to explain this in laymen's terms. He said that my brain processes information extremely fast, and that caused attention deficits. He went on to ask me if trying to stay focused on one topic was difficult. I agreed. He then asked me if it felt like I thought about too many things at one time, to which I also agreed.

This opened up a whole world of questioning from me. There was so much that I wanted to know about my brain injury. I wanted to know why I got massive adrenalin rushes. *Why do I get obsessed with ideas or thoughts? Why do*

I sometimes feel like there are several different versions of me?
I may have asked him that question a few times. I wanted
to know why I burned out so quickly. Of course, he told
me what every other doctor had said, "Your damaged
brain has to work twice as hard as it used to." I told him
that sometimes life seems to tire me out. I worried about
what was ahead of me and what further deficits this injury
may have in store for me. I wanted to know if it increased
my chances of having Parkinson's disease or Alzheimer's.
I told him nobody understands what I go through, and it
feels like there is no way of describing the side effects. I
think I freaked him out with all the questions, or maybe
with the rate of questions.

After I was finished, he answered as much as he could
but wanted me to seriously try to slow down my brain.
The concept of taking medication worried me. I thought
I might not see other problems if I was on medication.
The conversation got a bit frustrating because there was
no way I was going to take the medication, and I had
more to discuss with him. He stated that there may be
a possibility that I was bipolar. I just got up and walked
out. He mailed his results to me.

When we left there, Mary Beth stopped in front of
the building and said, "I have never heard you ask so
many questions. You really don't have anybody you can
talk to about this, do you?" I realized that I didn't have
anyone to talk to, because I thought that nobody would
understand what I was feeling. I admit, sometimes I
didn't know what I was becoming. It felt like there were
so many things I did well, yet maybe I didn't do enough

things well enough to manage my life. I started to wonder if everyone else saw a different version of me than I saw of myself.

I received the results from both tests a week later and brought them into work to discuss with George and the manager of Human Resources. The test results left nothing for me to explain, with the exception of some of the doctor's language. I gave a copy of the test results to George and asked him to please review them. I told him that both of us could meet with the Human Resource manager after he had read the results. I have to admit, it felt good to hand those results over to him because they were exactly what he did not want to see. I came back to his office a short while later and asked him if he was ready to head to the Human Resource manager's office. He replied, "There is no reason to discuss this with the Human Resource manager. Why don't we just leave this between us?"

What a shock! He did not want to discuss the test results. Still, I was glad I had tests performed. They made things better at work for a while, and I gained a greater understanding of my injury.

I tried to make adjustments after digesting these results. No, I was not ready to take the medicine the doctor recommended; however, I had a better understanding of what my deficits were and a comprehension of my strengths. Sometimes I felt like I was imagining all of this, and I had this dream that one miraculous visit to the doctor was going to clear it all up and I would be fine. Not this time, and not in this life.

I was getting so much better at how I portrayed myself. I spoke very well and at times came off as very detailed. This version of me made it difficult for someone to understand that I have or could have deficits. Too often there were times I came off as not very detailed, and I appeared to be disorganized and confused. Typically, this happened when I was stressed or overwhelmed; however, there were times when I appeared disorganized and confused for no other reason than I actually was. Another side of me came off as someone I didn't think was *me* at all. This version seemed to show up when I was at either end of the mood spectrum. Either I was pumped with adrenalin or burdened with depression. I hated the adrenalin version. I was all over the place personality-wise when this would happen. I honestly felt like someone took my body over. I was getting gradually better at controlling these drastic mood changes. What I learned to do was write myself a note that said *stay calm* or *be yourself.* I kept this note in my pocket, or sometimes I wrote it on the palm of my hand. I needed to do whatever it would take to stay on track. I now knew this was going to be a lifelong battle, and it was exhausting at times.

One change that occurred, and I cannot narrow down the year, was how I dealt with anger, specifically at work. I tried to lay a mental foundation for myself when it came to anger management, at least at work. I had this fear that if I lost my job, nobody would ever hire me, and my wife and kids would be in big trouble. I always told myself repeatedly when I thought I was entering a situation where I could lose my temper, *Stay calm. Stay calm.* One method I put into place that still works was to write down personal instructions to myself. I would write *stay calm* or *talk slow and don't interrupt.* And as always, I kept a picture of the kids in my pocket and pulled it out before meetings that I sensed were going to be less than pleasant. What my brain did, instead of letting the anger out, was the opposite—I would cry. I hated it. It wasn't exactly bundles of tears, it was more like a few would come out, just enough to cause a few water streaks on my face. There were times that I wish I just lost it, because the crying was humiliating. The crying was really the end result of not being able to say what I wanted. I knew how I was being judged, and there was nothing I could say or do about it. There were times I recall, and this still happens, where the tears would flow because I could not let the rage out. Yes, these injuries get stranger all the time. And maybe it is occurrences like this that form the platform for which I am judged.

The year 1998 should have ended on a good note at work. I was awarded the "Silver Eagle Award" for my accomplishments in sales. I also received the "Most Effective Manager to Plan" award from the corporate office. This award was the result of the national segment I managed attaining 120% of planned performance, which was an outstanding achievement given that the planned or expected effective percentage was only 88%.

As proud as I was for receiving these awards, George made sure that he rained on my parade. At the end of 1998, I finally sold an account that I had been assigned to for five years. It was the type of client where your chance of winning their business was a long shot at best. I always asked to remain assigned to this account because I liked the challenge of possibly winning the business, and I had established strong relationships with the client. I won the business right around Thanksgiving. This sale was the largest in my district and made me the number one candidate for a trip to Orlando, where the corporate office was going to recognize the top national sales of 1998.

George told me I was not going. I had made the sale after five years of hard work, but he had decided to send someone in my place. Now this angered me, as it would anyone. His reasoning was that since he was going to assign the account to someone else in 1999, the person assigned would go and accept the award. Neither I nor anyone else at work had ever heard of anything similar to this happening before. My belief was that George did not want me to be recognized in front of UPS hierarchy for what I had achieved. This was wrong, and everyone I worked with knew it. However, I had no idea where to turn to for advice, so I just moved on.

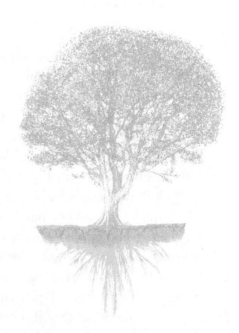

giving back and
moving on

After everything I had been through, both good and not so good, I realized I wanted to work with others who had brain injuries, specifically those in the early stages, which meant less than one year. I did not want to do this professionally of course, but I did want to be an example of what you can accomplish with a brain injury. Yes, I talk about all the issues I have, and sometimes being who I am contributes to those circumstances; however, there are so many challenges I have faced, and won, and will continue to win. I only have a fraction of the deficits that the doctors predicted for me. That being the case, I informed the faculty from my rehabilitation school that I would meet with anyone who would be interested. I also told the Brain Injury Association of Illinois of my intentions and that I would enjoy that type of interaction.

As luck would have it, UPS started a committee to which employees could submit, by department, charities that UPS would then consider donating money to. The committee was called the Community Involvement Committee. This started right after I had my first meeting with the Brain Injury Association of Illinois, and one of the items they had covered with me was a summer camp for those with brain injuries. This camp was located in Southern Illinois, and one reason I wanted to help was because so many inner-city kids who had suffered brain injuries did not have the financial means to attend. I wanted UPS to donate to this cause, and for weeks I pursued a contribution. Eventually, the donation was made, and in the summer of 1999 I had the privilege of presenting the Brain Injury Association of Illinois with a check that enabled four inner-city children the opportunity to attend the camp.

Work changed for me again in 1999. I was reassigned to the Key Segment, which presented me with a new group of challenges. I was the Area Sales Manager for nine account executives, and seven were relatively new. This was going to be a test for me since I would have to manage the activities of nine people who were inexperienced. It was different from the group I had managed before, where all I had to do was pave the road and assist them when needed. I was given a laptop computer. This was not one of my happier days. I felt a lot of anxiety wondering if I had the capacity to manage and learn a new technology at the same time. My plan boiled down to one path: honesty.

I had one-on-one meetings with all my account executives and told them the truth. What I explained to each of them individually was that I would struggle to remember a lot of what was told to me, so don't be offended if I forgot what you told me an hour or a day ago. I would remember small bites, but I didn't have the ability to remember big bites. If I tried to end our conversations short of what they had hoped, it was not because of lack of interest; it was because I had learned to stop when I realized there was no additional information that I was able to store. I also said that I would depend on them to assist me with certain items, and I would, in turn, assist them in areas I was strong in, primarily account management or client relations. They all understood, and I believe we worked well together.

UPS began testing us at this time on our product knowledge, and we had to have a ninety-five percent average or better to pass. I knew a lot about our products, but it was panic time for me because of the details they expected me to know. I had become skilled at knowing where to go to get answers as opposed to knowing the answers. There was another problem with the study guides we were given: since my TBI, I had difficulty reading a book. It was not that I couldn't read, I just couldn't remember what was on page two when I got to page three. I would have to read the same thing over and over again. There were times where I had to rely on a co-worker to help me get through the test. Don't get me wrong, I certainly was not in a "book of the month" club before my injury. I realized that I had short-term memory problems. When I read a newspaper, for example, I looked for the titles of articles that interested me and I focused on just enough of the article to comprehend the content.

One thing I always did well was let those who worked for me know that I was someone they could depend on, and I always wanted to know what was important to them outside of work. I would always stress that work is important, but not as important as enjoying and getting the most out of your life. We worked together just fine, and at the end of the year they graded me on what UPS calls an ERI, or Employee Relations Index. I received a ninety percent favorable, which was extremely high for this area. I hid my struggles quite well but continued to worry about how long I could hide them; however, I felt like I was winning the fight.

I spend a lot of time reviewing things I have done or said since I suffered my TBI. I look at certain situations and wonder if I could have handled them better. Sometimes I just shake my head and place an event into the crazy column. The following incident is one I am sure turned some heads and prompted laughter.

With the combination of my obsessive/compulsiveness and my belief that my story would be found interesting, this not-so-brilliant idea entered my mind. One day I was driving to work, and I heard the actor/director Harold Ramis on a local radio station. He was talking about movies he had done, such as *Animal House* and *Ghostbusters,* and I had what I thought was a great idea. Americans needed to see what brain injury victims went through, what we accomplished, and what we were capable of achieving in life. Since Harold had mentioned his office was in Illinois, I would take the story I wrote directly to him. Who you were or how famous you might be had no bearing on me. You were who you were. I never judged people by position or fame; I judged them by who they were, and to me, he seemed like a decent guy. I needed to find his office. He had mentioned his company's name, so all I had to do was find it.

I found the address within two hours, and what do you know, it was within driving range. I cleaned my story up, and the following week I took off from work in search of Harold Ramis. His office was in a well-to-do town in northern Illinois. I maneuvered my way around until I found it. It was on the second floor, and I had my selling hat on; I was going to walk out of there with Harold in complete agreement.

I knocked on the door, and his assistant answered. He was a young man in his early twenties, and I had talked to him earlier that week by phone. He remembered who I was, so he let me in. We were talking when I mentioned that I thought I was going to get pulled over because I wasn't driving a Mercedes. I heard someone chuckle in the office to my right, and out walked Harold Ramis. He had that Ramis smile on and said to his assistant, "Who's this guy?" in a funny sort of way. He was extremely nice and very down to earth; however, I was not very knowledgeable regarding the ways of Hollywood.

I tried to get in every word I could; I think I described my story as a mild comedic epic, which, of course, was a last resort. No sale. Nice guy, but no sale.

I was not stopping there. Someone had to make this story into a movie. Think about it: five guys head to a resort town in Wisconsin, and four come back. Who doesn't want to know what happened to the one who didn't come back? It had friendship, family, cops, good guys, bad guys, hospitals, rehab, court, violence, kids, bowling, corporate America, but it didn't have any sex.

I would not stop with Harold Ramis. I had another plan—Ron Howard. He seemed like a nice guy with a great résumé. He produced *A Beautiful Mind* with Russell Crowe, so he surely would like to produce *A Beautiful but Damaged Mind*. I called UPS in Connecticut to see if they knew where he lived, and if so, would they do me a small favor. They knew his address, and after I explained what I was trying to do, they agreed to deliver my story straight to his front door. *This can't miss,* I thought.

Turns out, they delivered it to his house, and I was told that his wife had signed for the delivery. All I had to do was wait for his letter or maybe a phone call.

I realize now that I was a bit out there...okay, a lot out there. I was convinced that my story as a movie was going to open the doors for those with brain injuries, and personally, I viewed it as my way of saying everything

I was afraid to tell those I knew did not believe or understand me. As I mentioned, a few things I look back on fall into the crazy column, and this one is a potential award winner. Everyone has dreams, though, and I was entitled to a few.

Every once in a while, I thought about what the doctor at the University of Illinois told me regarding medications that he thought would slow me down, or, as he put it, "slow my brain down." There were times I knew that too much ran through my mind, and the problem was, if it entered, it didn't leave. It was common for me to wake up at four o'clock in the morning and feel like I never went to sleep; my mind would start racing. There was only one logical thing to do: walk around the house, have some cookies with milk, and find something to do until I could crash again.

As I mentioned before, with a brain injury you often become more of what you once were. If you were impulsive prior to your brain injury, and I was, after you are extremely impulsive. I hate when it kicks in, because my filters are not very strong. For example, my cars have to be spotless. If it is 11:30 on a summer Thursday night, and I remember that my car is dirty, I will stop what I am doing and wash it. It will drive me crazy if I don't clean it. I do not have the ability to stop thinking about thoughts that enter my mind. I realize that everyone has experienced different games their minds play on them, and when I tell someone something that I experience, it is common for that person to say, "I have that all the time," or, "That happens to me too, and I don't have a brain injury." My problem is the extent to which I experience these conditions, the frequency I experience these conditions, and the number of different types of conditions I experience. These situations never stop; I just have to create a coping mechanism in order to deal with them. Creating coping mechanisms is much easier said than done.

Ron Howard's company, Imagine, sent me a letter! *I am a genius,* I thought. *My plan worked.* As I tore the letter open, I visualized what was written: "Your story floored me," or, "We are very interested." I started reading it, and I felt like a kid who had empty boxes under the tree at Christmas. It was a letter stating that I needed to send my treatment through a registered agent. There were only two in Chicago and I contacted both. One wanted me to find Jesus, and the other never sold a treatment. I had never lost Jesus, and the odds on the second were not very good, so that took care of that little idea.

Just to give you an insight into the movie concept, the truth is, I wanted to see the person I was after my injury. I have a fascination with the version of me that was born after 1992. For the most part, I have very little memory of what I was like during that first year. My brain was re-awakening, and I was just along for the ride. I had an idea that I would get this *understanding freedom* if what happened to me could be seen by all who were unaware of what brain injuries can do.

My UPS manager George was transferred in the fall of 1999 and replaced by an individual named Frank. When Frank arrived in Chicago, I handed him an envelope with my work history and wished him the best. I just did my job and kept my distance. Mary Beth told me not to discuss my brain injury, fearing Frank could think that I would not be able to do my job. I'm sure someone told him, but I was going to take Mary Beth's advice and not say a word.

A bowling alley opened in my town, and being that I enjoyed bowling, I investigated the possibility of joining a league. A Thursday night league was forming so I decided to join. At our first meeting, the topics of League President and League Secretary came up. The owner of the bowling alley volunteered to take the president's position; however, no one raised his hand for the secretary position. *How hard could that be?* I thought. *Collect the money each week and keep track of it, simple.* I raised my hand and was now the League Secretary.

I didn't link my struggle with numbers to the role of secretary. I always enjoyed that type of involvement, setting events up or just being part of something fun. I recruited some bowlers and my team was ready. When the league started and it was time for my "executive functions" deficit to kick in, I was immediately reminded that I had a TBI that impaired my ability to coordinate and keep track of twelve teams and bowling fees.

It was like someone turned the lights out. To the left was someone telling me, "We are fifteen dollars short," followed by someone asking me, "Can we hand in our money at the end of the game?" I had just volunteered for a nightmare. I was afraid to say anything so I just kept at it. I knew I could have handled it before my injury, no problem. My brain just could not process something so basic because of the many pieces, as simple as they may have been. I would have never linked my brain injury to something that I thought of as such a simple task.

I made it through the end of the season, and when it came time to figure out which team was short money or over, I was in "brain pain." It took me two full days to sort out that mess, and honestly none of it was right. Thank God it was a small league and I was cut some slack. Yes, I resigned my post. Before my injury, it was something I could have done without any difficulties. I did a great job of promoting the league, but that was the last time I volunteered for anything that required executive functions.

The year 2000 was right around the corner. The concern across America was "Y2K": computer systems crashing when December 31, 1999, gave way to January 1, 2000. If only I was so lucky. I thought, *If they crash, it is back to the old, somewhat simpler way, which is right up my alley.* I had learned a few things on my work computer, but I will admit that it was limited. Repeated exposure was my key to learning, so the more I used the computer the more familiar I became with it. I was going along okay at work; George was gone, so I didn't have to deal with him. Each November marked my new year. I began to mark the years as the time period since I had almost died. It felt like a different life at times, so I guess it made sense. With each new year, I would celebrate the strides I had made, and at the same time consider the long road ahead of me. However, something unexpected happened at this time and I marveled at the experience.

A friend of mine at work, Sandy, approached me one Monday morning in early 2000 and explained how a good friend had crashed his car into a tree over the weekend and was in a coma. She described his injuries and what his family had been told by the doctors. It sounded similar to what my family had heard after my injury. Sandy asked if I would go with her to visit her friend and his family when the time was right, and I agreed. It was strange how much I wanted to do this.

He was at Northwestern Memorial Hospital and was beginning rehabilitation at the Rehabilitation Institute of Chicago. I remember walking in his room; his family was there, and after I introduced myself and explained all I had been through, his mother cried and hugged me. I realized that I was a strong ray of hope; it was a beautiful feeling for such a sad, unfortunate experience. As I approached him lying in his bed I observed the way he appeared and tried to compare it to how I was. He had a patch over one eye for the same reason as I once did, paralyzed on the same side that I was. The victim was in his early thirties, a business professional who was married and had two small children. His accident was a fluke. He had taken his new sports coupe for a ride on Sunday morning, lost control, and hit a tree. I asked if I could talk to him. I recall trying to imagine exactly what he was able to comprehend about what was going on. There really is nothing as unimaginable or confusing as a brain injury. I knew from experience that what I said would be forgotten in a matter of seconds, but it was important to him that we talked, and it was important to me.

I kept in contact with this new member of the "every 21 seconds club" for a few years. We would have lunch once in a while, and he would express the challenges he had at home and how frustrating it was. His short-term memory was damaged, so he struggled with that as well as the frustration of trying to get used to his new life. He had problems at home, mostly centered around his relationship with his wife, which is all too common. I told him that my recommendation would be to talk about the problems, try to work together, and avoid getting to the point where his temper would be lost. We covered the same topics every time we met. Mary Beth talked to his wife. I believe his wife appreciated and took hope from listening to her experience. At times, I'm sure it must have felt like no one understood. Unfortunately, any help we could give was not enough, and the couple eventually divorced. Prior to the brain injury, they were perceived as the perfect couple.

When my brain injury occurred, Mary Beth did not have someone who could sympathize with what she was going through or give her insight into what to expect. Ironically, our family's exposure to a TBI was through my dad's only brother, Pat. At the time of my injury, my dad was recovering from his stroke and really could not provide insight into his brother's TBI. My mom always described Pat's post-TBI life with one word: terrible. Pat was a Chicago police officer assigned to the motorcycle division. He had picked up his three-wheel Chicago

Police Department motorcycle from the repair shop and headed for Lake Shore Drive. He was traveling at a high rate of speed when the wheels flew off. It appeared the repair shop had neglected to tighten the lug nuts on the wheels. Pat was wearing a helmet; however, his head, as well as his body in general, had hit the pavement so hard, and so fast, that he suffered massive injuries.

Pat survived but was left with serious physical and cognitive deficits. There was minimal therapy in 1968, so he was pretty much on his own. Pat spent six months in the hospital before going home. Like eighty percent of couples in which one of the two suffers a TBI, Pat and his wife divorced and he lived alone for his remaining years. Pat, like me, had desperately wanted to return to work, and the Chicago Police Department found a way to accommodate Pat's wish. He was given a desk job, but more important to Pat was that he had his uniform on. A squad would pick him up every day and drive him to work, where he would sit at his desk. Outside of his kids, it was all he really had.

I always heard stories about how Pat was before his accident, but the only version I knew was the post-brain injury version. I remember going to see him when I was just a kid, or years later when he would stop by my dad's house just to talk. He died ten years after his accident as a result of complications from his injuries. My dad once told me, years before my TBI, that because Pat suffered so much after his accident, he wondered if it may have been a blessing if Pat had passed when it happened. Thank God he told me that before my injury.

The opportunities for me to become an inspiration to other TBI victims continued to crop up, unfortunately. I say unfortunately because for me to become a ray of hope, someone else had to suffer a brain injury. However, it was still something I truly enjoyed doing. I always felt as if it gave me the ability to take something that was a negative and turn it into a positive. The feeling I would get from making a difference in someone's life was incredible.

The one issue that is consistent with the majority of TBI victims is a severe reduction in self-confidence. It is torn to shreds from the injury, and then life's experiences seem to chip away at what remains. I know that at times I take things too personally and assume that the brain injury is the reason why these unfortunate situations occur. Too some extent that is true; however, what I am dealing with is mine to deal with, and nobody else can see it. The more normal you appear, the more difficult it is for anyone to assume that your shortfalls are from your injury. I once had someone tell me, after I was explaining the details of one of my deficits, "You, you're fine. You drive, you work, so you're fine." If only it was that simple.

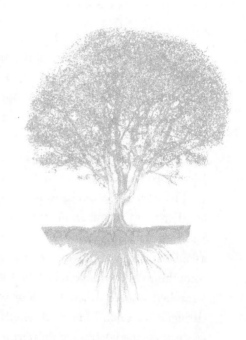

getting closer
to the fire

As the year 2000 was under way, I was given some good news at UPS. I was asked to report to my division manager's office. Frank had been here a few months and was trying to adjust to the new position. Frank had told me that the decision was made to promote me to National Account Manager. He didn't tell me who specifically made this decision and I really didn't care. What was great about this position for me was that I would be able to focus on a few large accounts, and I was confident I would be successful. I only had to worry about myself, not managing others. Another bonus would be that I would have an assistant to help me keep track of things. I was told to pack up my desk because I was being moved in the next week or two. I called home to tell Mary Beth. I was absolutely ecstatic.

The next three weeks went by, and Frank never said another word to me about the position, so I figured he just lost track. I made my way down to his office and asked when I was moving to my new position. I knew something was wrong; I just had a bad feeling. When I reached Frank's office, the door was open and he was sitting at his desk. I knocked quietly and told him that I was wondering when I would start my new sales position. It appeared that he did not want to discuss the subject. Maybe he felt uneasy about it. At first, he was silent; then he quietly said, "Truth is, someone stopped you from getting that position, and you really don't want to know why they stopped it or who stopped it." *Well*, I thought, *why don't you just punch me in the head while you are at it?*

"It's the brain injury, isn't it?" I responded. Frank didn't deny it, and with that I left. My history in sales justified my promotion to the National Account Manager position. *How could someone do this, and why did I have to find out this way?* If there was a legitimate reason for reversing the decision, why wasn't it explained to me? What did Frank mean by "you don't want to know who or why?" If it had nothing to do with my brain injury, why would he not tell me the actual reason?

I am not sure how I could have done a better job of proving myself. I won five sales awards the previous three years, so why was it handled this way? Some years later, I was told that the manager who decided to reverse my promotion made the following statement to a mutual friend when asked why I was not in sales: "He (me) has issues." That statement is open to individual interpretation, but from my perspective it was a direct reference to my brain injury. The experience was humiliating. For three weeks, I told those who reported to me that I would be training my replacement because I was finally awarded the position I had earned and that would best utilize my abilities. Now I had to tell them someone had stopped it. The refusal of Frank to give me an explanation was the most humiliating part.

This was the start of the most difficult years since my accident. To make matters worse, I had a grand mall seizure in the summer of 2000. There was a study done in 1992, the same year as my injury, that found that individuals with head trauma were twelve times as likely as the general population to suffer seizures. Seizures like the one I had are common immediately following an injury to the brain or may develop months, or in some cases years, after the initial injury. Generally speaking, the risk of seizures is directly related to the severity of the brain injury. The chances of having a seizure fluctuate based on the severity of the injury. When the seizure occurred, my neighbors were with Mary Beth and me on a sunny summer morning, and then lights out. My head snapped back like a rubber band, and I collapsed. This scared everyone who saw it. I never remembered the other seizures I had experienced, since they were all within a month after my injury. I didn't go to the hospital, because I was afraid of what they would tell me. I just prayed it was a fluke and that I would not have another one.

In September of 2000, I was removed from my sales manager position and transferred to marketing. This was a shock, as I never thought that marketing was in my future. Frank called me out of a meeting and told me I was being assigned to the marketing side of the house. Sales were what I did extremely well; however, I remember thinking, due to how this new assignment was presented so negatively to me, that something was up. The next week I was invited to have lunch with my new division manager, Ron, who was domiciled in the western Chicago suburbs. He handed me a written description of the job, told me to learn a specific computer program, and wrapped it up nicely by saying, "Don't call me. I'll call you." I was told to stay in the building and communicate via e-mail.

A month later, I was asked to be the subject of a newspaper article, which coincidentally was located in the same town where my new manager's office was located. The article was titled "Local Man Battles Against Brain Injury." The Brain Injury Association of Illinois had recommended me to the newspaper, and I was glad to do it. I hoped that maybe someone at UPS would read the article and maybe, just maybe, ask me about my disability. The article discussed how I compensated for my deficits. It talked about how I managed my job at work, and it had quotes from specialists at the institute where I had my rehabilitation. Of course, the comments were directed at me and brain injury patients in general. Nobody at UPS read it, or maybe they did and never said a word. I sent the article to Ron. He just sent it back a few days later. I don't really know why I did that; maybe I thought everyone at UPS should be as proud of me for being so far ahead of what the doctors had predicted. Live and learn: I realize now my brain injury meant nothing to Ron and I was wrong to assume he would care. He never brought it up to me and I wondered if sending him that article about my brain injury would come back to haunt me.

My new position appeared to lack a clear definition. I was located in the building where I had been a sales manager, yet I had little to no contact with Ron, my manager. I felt as though they had no idea what to do with me and figured they would let me gather dust until I quit.

Maybe there was something I didn't see or realize about myself. Why had I recovered so well and been so successful under Thomas Farrell and Shawn O'Leary, but in recent years it felt like a roadblock had been placed in my career path? One step forward, two steps back, but I wasn't going away.

One thing that UPS, or any company who has an employee with a brain injury, should do is ask the person a few simple questions, such as: *What do you struggle with, or what areas pose significant problems for you?* They all knew I had this injury. It was on my medical history, and every time I was moved, my prior manager would tell the new one, "He has a brain injury." I hoped they worded it that way. I know it was discussed, because at some point it was always brought to my attention. By asking these questions, a company can find out what our strengths and weaknesses are. I knew dealing with me at times could be frustrating. I admitted that. Yes, I often forgot some of what I was told; yes, my mind raced, making it hard for me to stay focused; yes, I could have difficulty with executive functions, and the list goes on. However, I could still do a multitude of tasks quite well; I'd proven that. The chances of me doing a cognitive task successfully increased when that task fell in the range of things I still did well. I was determined, persistent, and I gave everything I did a hundred percent effort. And I was not a quitter.

I bring up UPS a lot. It was and still is a part of my life. It is responsible for some of my best memories, and unfortunately it is also responsible for a lot of disappointments. This company at one time was like a family, but that seemed to disappear. I grew up there, so maybe that is why I harbor such resentment at how I was treated simply because I have a brain injury. However, flip the coin over, and I will tell you there is not another company on earth that would have given me the opportunities I received from UPS. I am not by any means trying to point fingers; I am just trying to highlight areas of ignorance so that maybe my story will help others who suffer from the same injury. Sure, my experiences were hard on me; however, I know my experiences may pale in comparison to what other traumatic brain injury survivors encounter.

I noticed that how I behaved or reacted around my family members differed from how I may have been perceived outside my immediate family. I never really understood why I was this way. However, it is common among TBI survivors to feel or act this way. Inside my house there were times I felt on edge, always obsessing about what was going on with my life outside of the home. I know now that the cause of this behavior was from my lack of control over situations outside of the house, predominately at work. No matter how I was treated or made to feel, in my mind there was nothing I could do about it. Sure, I could have left the company, but without a college degree and with my medical history, my choices were extremely limited. I felt trapped in my life.

My injury caused me to be a bit paranoid at times. I never knew what others were thinking, and I know now that talking about my injury may not have been a good move. I don't know why I chose to speak about my brain injury. I believe it was my way of dealing with it. I wonder why I thought anyone would care. Chances are, it gave those I discussed the injury with a perception that I was different, or they assumed I was lying or exaggerating something they couldn't see or understand. A former president of the Brain Injury Association of Illinois told me that I am a Catch-22. She said that because I have no visible physical limitations and I carry myself well, I am always going to have problems with co-workers understanding my deficits. What can't be seen, can't be understood. She hit the nail on the head.

Welcome to the land of impulsivity. I could tell you about all the impulsive things I have done since the injury, but I will limit the list to a few select items. In the spring of 2001, I was close to out of my mind trying to find that one item to look forward to. Work was just a frustrating "mind game," and other parts of life were stagnant. This was always a perfect recipe for me to go buy or do something impulsive.

A co-worker asked me to take a ride with him to Perillo BMW in downtown Chicago. This co-worker had wanted a BMW for years. He was logical about his purchase, or future purchase. Unfortunately, he brought me with him. We walked in to the dealership; he went one way, and I went the other. About ninety minutes later, he had a brochure, and I had a receipt for a brand new BMW 323. I took off work the following day to pick up the car and bring it home.

When Mary Beth pulled up and saw my black BMW sitting in the driveway, she just smiled and said, "Nice car, Bri." No shock at all. I bought a cover for the car and waxed it every month. I loved that car. On a side note, I felt like the car was made for me, because the Brain Injury Association of America had declared BMW one of the best cars made for reducing the chances for brain injuries in the event of a collision. I thought, *Hey, I certainly couldn't afford another injury, so this is the perfect car for me.* You use whatever means you can to justify impulsiveness.

The rest of 2001 was somewhat uneventful with the exception of being transferred from my current work site to the regional office. I cannot begin to explain just how disappointed I was with the move. Working in this setting was a mix between a library and a funeral home lobby. I didn't fit in at all. I'm not one to easily adjust to sitting still in front of a computer, especially after my accident. Like I said before, I am not a computer person, and I just don't have the patience needed for sitting still. Of course, I figured out that the more water I drank, the more reasons I had for getting up and taking a walk to the men's room.

I never went to lunch with anyone; for some reason it felt like an escape to go to lunch alone. Since my accident, I seem to enjoy being alone at times. Whether it is in my car or in a room, I like being by myself and thinking. Normally, I dream about the way I wish things were, and I don't mean family-wise, I mean life in general. I think about my injury too much. I miss the way my life felt before the injury, and more specifically, I miss loving every aspect of my life. I would think about things in my future that I could look forward to. In the song "In My Room," the Beach Boys' Brian Wilson wrote, "In my room I lock out all my worries and my fears." Sometimes that line fits. There are times life feels like it is going too slow, and there are other times when life feels like it is taking too long.

The end of 2001 was right around the corner, and the tension at work was just a hair shy of severe. I knew the whole thing was going to come to a head, and I think mentally I was ready. It was the calm before the storm. One of the work events that seemed like a "take a hint" moment went something like this: Ron had asked me to stop by his manager's office so the two of them could give me direction on a few tasks. Each one was throwing tasks at me like Frisbees at a show dog. I didn't take in a word they were saying.

After the meeting ended, I had to say something. I told them I could not keep pace with what the two of them had just covered, and I would like to discuss a potential tool that would assist me. I told them that I had a brain injury, which I knew they were aware of, and I had some deficits in regards to retaining new information. I had recent medical reports that outlined methods or tools that would be helpful during meetings. One of the tools I mentioned was a recorder. This was a recommended coping mechanism, and I said that it would be truly helpful in my completing work-related tasks. I said, "I don't want anything special, just a chance to meet your expectations." They reply was an instantaneous "no." There were no counter proposals such as, "Maybe we can review your doctor's suggestions," or, "I am not comfortable with recorders. Maybe we could try an alternate method." There was nothing other than a straight-to-the-point "no." Believe me, admitting that I can't do something is not that easy, and what I was trying to do was compensate for a deficit that I could not control.

The storm was right around the corner, and the strange part was, I knew the path I was going to have to take. That path was going on disability, which I did not want to do;

however, it was either that or risk going absolutely crazy. I had conversations with my primary physician, and he said that he would support my disability because he felt I was one letter shy of a breakdown. He was right.

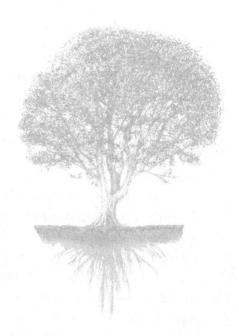

the missing piece

The house in Lake Geneva, Wisconsin, my four friends and I had stayed at that November weekend was torn down a few years after my injury. Mary Beth's mother, Sandra, and her sister, Kathleen, had built two new homes on the land. Kathleen was turning forty that first weekend in 2002, and we were invited to her mom's house for a birthday surprise party.

On the way to the party, I told Mary Beth that I couldn't see the tension at work lasting longer than another week. It just seemed like a bomb was going to go off, and I guess I was ready for it. I felt like the tension of knowing that something unfortunate was right around the corner seemed more harmful than whatever was going to happen. Stress eats me up, and this was killing me. I knew what Ron, my manager at UPS, wanted and I began to think that I was ready to face whatever he had planned.

As we drove that January weekend, I kept thinking about the first meeting I had with Ron and the other individuals I would work with in the marketing segment. I really didn't know anyone in the marketing department. What was disturbing was after that meeting when Dan, one of my new co-workers, said, "Did you rain on his parade?" I didn't know what to say. Just then another person in the room said, "For some reason he doesn't like you." There wasn't a reason for Ron to dislike me, at least none that I was aware of. I had met Ron before, but our limited interactions were all about business. I tried to figure out a way to erase it all from my mind, for a few days at least. However, I kept thinking that sending him the article about my brain injury, which outlined some of my deficits, may have been a very bad idea. Mary Beth always cautioned me about bringing up my brain injury. She was afraid it could negatively affect how I was judged or evaluated, and advised me to keep it quiet. Now I suppose it was possible that Ron had been told by others whom I had worked for that I had a short-term memory deficit or could become confused when given too much information. Ron may also have been told that I could sometimes have difficulty following instructions. Perhaps he was lead to believe that he was given a "lemon."

When we arrived at Mary Beth's mom's house, I let her and the kids out of the car and repeated what I had done every time I had been there since my injury. I told them all, "I will be right back." I drove two blocks to the bar where the injury occurred.

As always, I parked across the street and stared at where I was found, face down in the street. I guess my reason for going to that site was always the same. I wondered what life would have been like if I had left two minutes later that night. I know that as lucky as I was to have survived, almost ten years later too many parts of my life were not in order. For some reason, I thought that a lost memory from that night would come back to me. I just wanted the missing pieces of my life back. I lost so much time those first few years. I stayed there for about ten minutes and went back to the house.

We had been at the party for a while, and I was doing my usual small talk and walking around. I was introduced to a neighbor of Mary Beth's sister who was originally from Chicago. The guy seemed nice enough and quite relaxed, as he had been at the party for a while. We had been talking about nothing specific when I asked him how long he had been living in Lake Geneva, what he did for a living, and other trivial questions. We got through all of the small talk, so I asked him if he remembered the incident at the bar up the road. I gave him the year and a few general points, nothing too specific. I was so hoping he would say yes—it was a small town—and I knew there

had to be a Lake Geneva version of what happened. His
eyes lit up.

"You mean the fight at that bar?"

"Yeah, the fight," I replied.

He continued. "Well, the guy from Chicago died a
few years after that fight, and I think he was the brother
of the lady who lives here."

"He was?" I replied.

"Yeah, I think he was," he said, "'cause she never talks
about him. I work with the brother-in-law of the guy
who killed him."

I had struck gold! This was so fascinating that I could
not wait to hear how I had died.

"Do you know how he died?" I asked.

"Yes, yes, I do," he replied. "What happened was this
guy, Nick Smith, was kicked out of the bar for throwing
a drink on someone. Well, he went back in to get his
wife and he ended up hitting a few people on the way
back in. I think one was a lady who worked there. Well
some of the people working at the bar chased Nick out
of the bar and they started beating on him. When Nick
got up he was pissed, and he saw the guys from Chicago
walking out of the place and he just lost it and punched
one of them in the back of the head. When the guy from
Chicago went down, he finished him off with his steel-
toed boots."

"Finished him off?" I asked.

"Yah, he kicked him in the head a few more times,
and that is what eventually killed the guy."

"How well do you know your friend from work?" I asked.

"I know him as a friend, not a close one."

Then he proceeded to tell me how he had seen Smith a few years ago, and he had not been the same since it had happened. *Well, that makes two of us,* I thought. I looked at him and grinned, because I knew what I was going to tell him would cause his jaw to drop.

"You know, the guy from Chicago never died."

"How do you know that? Do you know him?" he asked.

"Yes, I do, and the reason I know he never died is because you're talking to him," I said.

His color suddenly disappeared, and he looked like someone had just spray-painted his face white. He stared at me and said, "Oh, I am so sorry. I didn't know it was you."

He started to get teary-eyed, so I said, "Don't worry about it. I'm glad you told me some things I never knew."

He kept saying how sorry he was, which was kind of funny, because there was nothing to be sorry about. I mean, he thought Smith had killed his neighbor's brother, and our little conversation had changed all that. I wonder if he ever told Smith's brother-in-law about our conversation.

With that, I excused myself and went upstairs to tell Mary Beth. If you recall, early on the doctors had said that there was too much damage to my brain to be just a fist to the back of the head and something else must have happened. A little more than nine years later, another missing piece of the puzzle came together. I pulled Mary Beth aside and told her about the conversation. Mary Beth had this look on her face as if it hurt more knowing that my head was used as a soccer ball.

I will admit that for the first time since the accident I actually had anger toward the guy who had changed my life, if, in fact, what I had been told was true. I was angry that he may have bragged to people that he kicked me in the head while I was down. It wasn't something I would brag about. But the anger was short-lived; I was strangely relieved that after all these years I knew the truth. All I ever wanted was to know exactly what had happened. I always asked everyone to tell the truth. It just made it more understandable for me. Outside of Mary Beth, I never bothered to tell anyone about that conversation. I guess it seemed to matter to me, and I didn't think anybody else would care.

Thursday, January 10, 2002, I was stationed in the back of the building at work, near the rear exit. There was someone who sat about fifteen feet away from me, but nobody ever sat near me. I may not have been the sharpest knife in the drawer, but even I figured it out what was going on. It appeared someone had asked a female co-worker to sit next to me and see if I used the company phone or computer for anything non-work related. I knew what she was doing there, and I went about my day. I didn't care either way. I never brought a cell phone into work, so there were times I had to use the work phone to call home. My daughter had incurred some front-end damage to her car, and I had to use the phone to check on the status of the work. That was all she needed to hear. I left for lunch, and when I came back all of her belongings were gone. My manager, Ron, asked me to grab my laptop and meet him in his office.

He started by going through my laptop, e-mail by e-mail. He would ask the status of every e-mail if it didn't have our company name after it. There were a few that were from former co-workers who had e-mailed me a Merry Christmas wish a few weeks earlier. He asked who they were, and I answered. He would then ask, "Did you reply?" My answer was yes, to which he said, "That is a company violation." He then asked if I had recently used the phone for non-work-related calls. I said yes and explained the car situation. He then told me to leave the building and call in the next day to check on my employment status.

Funny, walking out that door seemed like a relief. When I got in my car, I made two calls: one to my doctor and one to a friend in management at UPS. I made an appointment to see my doctor in the morning. The friend from work was someone I trusted, and I let him know what had just happened. I started my car, slipped in a favorite CD, and off I went. For a brief moment I felt relieved, though I knew in my heart the rest of the year could be torture.

I went home and took my suit off, which I had always hated wearing. I drove directly to where Mary Beth worked and told her that the bomb had gone off. She was very calm about it, as was I.

The following day I went to my doctor's office and

explained what had happened. I always gave him updates so he was not shocked. He proceeded to put me on disability for extreme stress. That information was faxed over to UPS. The following Monday I was to report to the Employee Relations manager to discuss what had transpired. His name was Ted. To say that I was ready for this meeting was an understatement.

I arrived at Ted's office and we were joined by Ron. First, Ron gave his reasons for his dissatisfaction with my job. They were written on one page of a Franklin planner. Here were a few of his concerns: bad date on an expense account, casual wear on a non-casual day, bad vocabulary on a newsletter I had written (he told me that I was a terrible writer. I guess he won't be reading this book), and that I had used a company copier to make a one-page copy of a personal document. I did not deny any of Ron's accusations. When Ron was finished, I asked, "That's it?" I was not intimidated, not this time.

I laid out what I had prepared, which was about thirty-five pages of material. I had documented everything, just as I was taught in rehabilitation. Included in my documentation was a three-page letter to the CEO of UPS describing in detail what I had been put through since my TBI. Along with the letter to the CEO were documents outlining how I had been treated. I also included doctor's reports, my individual company reviews, career highlights since my TBI, my resume outlining my UPS career, and the University of Illinois neurological test results from two years prior. I read my letter to the CEO aloud, and as I reached the end of the letter Ron became angry and Ted asked him to leave the room. After the meeting, I went home to begin my unscheduled vacation.

I had a plan for the time I was going to be off. The plan was no haircuts, daily visits to the health club, meet with the doctor as prescribed, remodel a few close friends' houses, and try to figure out my future. As I mentioned earlier, Ron called me to tell me that I was not being paid during my absence. According to Ron and someone from Human Resources he had on the line with him, I was not being paid because the insurance company had denied my disability.

It was denied was because my psychiatrist had stated in her reports that I was neatly dressed and properly groomed. Since I was neatly dressed and properly groomed, all disability pay was denied, regardless of what the doctor had documented and recommended. Incredibly, the insurance company believed that brain injury survivors are incapable of dressing properly and practicing good personal hygiene. How could they be sure someone hadn't dressed me and properly groomed me?

The visits with the psychiatrist proved to be insightful. For weeks we would talk, and she had one major suggestion: quit UPS and do something different. I never wanted to do that. As a company, UPS had been so good to me. I reminded her that I had four kids, and I really did not want to leave. That company was all I knew. As always, I believed that one day a magic wand would be waved over me and life at work and home would return to the way it was before my brain injury.

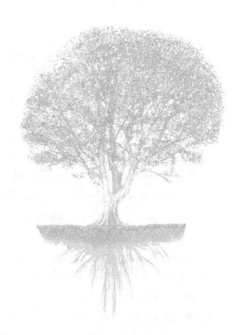

the collapse

Before we head back to Thanksgiving 2002, I would like to declare that brain injuries are as mysterious to me as maybe they are to you. I have spent years trying to live with one, and at times I tried to pretend my injury didn't exist. There are days, based on the circumstances life has asked you to face, that you are at the mercy of your brain injury. There have been times where I would review in my mind the way I reacted, or the way I wished I would have reacted, to certain situations and realized I would have handled things differently before my injury.

Conversely, there have been difficult situations where I felt as though I handled certain challenges or situations quite well. I recall times where the pressure of all that was going on in my life, specifically negative situations, dropped me to my knees. I know at times I took on more than I should have. However, I do believe I faced a lot of negative, stressful situations that I never should have had to deal with. As I look back, I remember how hard I tried to prove that I was okay after my injury. I would try so hard to convince the therapists and doctors that the damage to my brain was just a brief setback. I know now that returning to work was my way of proving that I was fine. I cannot expect people to understand how "tricky" a brain injury can be, and I know that as long as these injuries continue they will be misunderstood.

The last ten years has been an interesting decade for me. I have accomplished virtually everything my family was told I would never be able to do, as well as some things that may have been in my best interest to avoid. I have tried to be accepted by others for who I am today. I never hid the fact that I have this injury, and never understood why some people treated me differently because of it. For some reason, I always felt that going back to the life I had was a moral victory for me, and it was even more satisfying to let others know that I had triumphed over a traumatic brain injury that was supposed to shut me down.

I have covered how the injury affected my home life, personal life, and of course my life at work. Mary Beth will not talk about my brain injury unless I ask, or I act in a way that I never would have pre-injury. Obviously, I had to ask her a lot of questions regarding who I was or who I became after my injury, and some answers were immediate and some answers took more time. One piece of information she recently told me was one of the most interesting things ever revealed about my injury.

Mary Beth said that although I shouldn't have returned to work, or at least not when I did, it was therapeutic for me because the better I felt about myself the less obvious were my deficits. Although there were difficult times the first few years, I was provided a positive and supportive work environment by those I initially had reported to. Mary Beth said when those individuals moved on and I was working for managers who did not provide the same type of understanding and support, my recovery actually regressed. Deficits that may have been dormant came streaking back, in some cases erasing the progress I had made.

Brain injuries surface in ways where it is difficult for the average person to realize actions or statements made are a direct result of the injury. You may appear to act irrationally or in ways that seem out of line. You may distance yourself from friends and family. You may sleep for hours on end; conversely, you may experience insomnia. Of course, you may, as I have indicated, experience emotional outbursts that would ordinarily never occur in the absence of brain injury. What Mary Beth pointed out made so much sense, although it was obvious, but I never realized it at the time. She said I was making such great progress, and when the work environment changed, I took two steps backwards. It was a gradual regression.

There were also deficits that showed up for the first time, after years of being doormant, under unfavorable conditions. Negative situations would be amplified tenfold because of my brain's inability to properly focus when stressed. I could not stop how rapidly thoughts would run through my brain; it was nothing shy of indescribable torture. You would have to experience it to believe it. The sad part was I tried as best I could to just keep it in, and when I couldn't do that anymore I would have complete shutdown. I believe Mary Beth's observation were dead-on accurate.

Although I wish I had not been so consumed with trying to get back to my former life, I can't change history. However, of all the years since my injury, the year 2002 was the worst. Writing a poem about attending your own funeral is not on anyone's list of normal things to do. I really wanted to escape everything that was going on. Life, my life, felt completely out of my control. Everything became an unwanted job that year. Getting up, getting dressed, eating, being a dad, being a husband, being alive, all of that became a fight. I don't believe I ever wanted to die; I just wasn't sure that the life was at all like it should be.

Since my injury, I tried to do those things that validated my recovery. While I was doing that, I had tried too relentlessly for acceptance in every aspect of my life. When I failed, I took that failure too hard. There were two main parts of my life, first my family and then my job. I felt like I was failing on the family side, but my failure was directly related to the situation at work. The combination was, at best, lethal. Life became something it was never supposed to be.

Back to Thanksgiving morning, 2002. How did this day ever happen? How can life get to a point where you don't even recognize it? As much as company on Thanksgiving is welcome, typically you would not invite the police and their friends, the paramedics. I had a feeling that this day was going to come, but I didn't think it would be so dramatic.

After the police and the paramedics left, I went downstairs, checked on Jim, and made my way to the kitchen. As Mary Beth and the kids entered, I was busy staring out the window, not ready to turn around. Eventually, I turned, and there they were, sitting at the table. I looked at all of them, the little ones, the older two, and Mary Beth. They just looked confused. I really didn't know what to say, so I decided to leave for a while. I took a drive and returned twenty minutes later.

When I got home, I tried as best as I could to comprehend the past year. I told Mary Beth that I was going to move out, at least until the upcoming doctor visit, which was only three short weeks away. I said that I thought it would be best for all of us if I left. Not a lot was said regarding my proposal, not even, "You could stay, but you have to sleep in the shed." We decided to tackle the issue later in the day.

I had another problem heading my way; the family Thanksgiving dinner was being held at my house. The good side was the guests were limited to my mom and my sister's family. It was too late to turn back, so we decided to act our way through it. We asked the kids not to mention a word of what had happened.

I went upstairs to shower and get the blood out of my hair that was there from my hitting the coffee table. I know what you are thinking: *Sounds like one bizarre holiday.* I agree. Thank God I still had a healthy head of hair and was able to hide the damage. My mom would snap if she saw my scalp. Of course, she would faint if she knew how I had cut my head.

Everyone arrived on time, and we weren't five minutes into our meal when my five-year-old daughter, Jenna, said, "There was an ambulance at our house today."

Mary Beth quickly responded, "Jenna, just eat your food!"

Jenna added softly, "The police were here, too."

Everyone knew that something had happened, but everyone chose to believe that Jenna was just saying something silly. Jim looked at me and we both smiled, which made the situation a bit easier to deal with.

Later that day, after everyone had left, I told Jim how sorry I was about the last few months, and especially about today. He said, "We all feel bad for you, Dad. You seem to be struggling all the time." That was the nicest thing anyone could have said to me. That Thanksgiving Day was the only time Jim and I had ever experienced something like that, we always got along so well. Sure, we had typical father/son disagreements, but that was it.

When the topic of me moving out for a while came up later, I was asked not to.

What happened to me was a breakdown due to what was going on in my life mixed in with a traumatic brain injury. Everything I spoke about in Chapter One, and what I have reviewed here, was the result of a mental or nervous breakdown. The sad part was I tried to just keep going, and we all paid the price for that. It went on for so long, I lost the ability to identify how I had psychologically deteriorated.

The four-day holiday weekend was over and Monday morning arrived. The only thing on my mind was trying to figure out how to tell Ron that I needed to take a few days off for testing regarding my brain injury. I was intimidated when it came to mentioning my brain injury. Earlier in the year when I had returned from disability, I had been told by Earl, the Employee Relations Manager, to never mention my brain injury or disability again. This being the case, I had to figure something out.

Due to the nature of our business we were extremely busy at Christmas time, and you were never supposed to take time off unless you passed away. Even then, you needed a doctor's note. So I did the most logical thing: I left my manager, Ron, and his manager, Tony, a voicemail indicating that on December 17 I had to go to the hospital for testing. I did not say what I was to be tested for; I just said *tested.* My immediate manager never responded. Tony did respond, and he told me via voicemail to be sure that I did not miss the appointment, which actually made me feel somewhat better. Outside of all that had gone down and the bad feelings that existed, Tony responded promptly and professionally. I knew there was nothing he would have liked better than a resignation notice from me, but outwardly he stayed professional.

I was counting the days until I was able to meet with the doctor. His name was Dr. Kay, considered one of the best post-brain injury doctors in the Midwest. Mary Beth was going with me to the appointment.

At work I was told to organize a *Toys for Tots* campaign. This campaign was sponsored by the U.S. Marines. I was supposed to gather up volunteers at work to make pickups at banks where the toys had been dropped off throughout Chicago and the suburbs. This was to take place on the December 16, the day before my doctor's appointment.

For some reason Ron, who had limited knowledge of the city, assumed that we could get all the toy pickups in a day even though the banks closed at five p.m. Everybody else involved had a different opinion, so we figured we would do all we could and hope for the best. We kept in mind that it was a volunteer effort and the Marines who were in charge appreciated everything that we did.

Things at home were better, at least better than Thanksgiving. Every day closer to the appointment gave me a little more comfort. I was trying so hard to make it to that day. I know I was a mess, but I had something in front of me that, at the time, meant everything to me. The impact a TBI has on someone is indescribable. Sadly, the only way to comprehend the damage is to experience it yourself...Correction to that statement: I think living with someone who has suffered a TBI gives you a pretty good indication of how powerful an injury it can be. I really tried to believe that this was going to be a turning point for me.

On December 16, I had someone with me from work on my route, and we ran from morning until night. We covered the west, east, south, and northern parts of the city. We fell two pick-ups shy of the thirty-something pick-ups they had asked us to do. When we showed up at the Marine base that night, they were thrilled that we had finished as many as we had, and they would run down the street in the morning and get the two we missed.

December 17 was the day I had been waiting for so desperately. I really felt like this was it. It had been ten years since my injury, and I was not going to hold anything back. There I was back in the hospital with Mary Beth, and my plan was to just lay it all out on the table. We were there first thing in the morning, and I was in a very strange but laid-back mood. As I was introduced to the doctor, the same thought that I have every time I meet a doctor raced through my mind: *I wonder if he will think I am normal.* I know that sounds strange, but I always wondered how difficult it was for brain injury doctors to view you as a normal person. You wish you could bring in the original version of yourself so he could compare the two. It would be like parking two identical cars next to each other that look the same but run just a bit differently, and the doctor's job would be to check under the hood to find the problem.

First, he went over my medical records relating to the past ten years, and then we talked. I told him everything

I possibly could, and it felt good to let it all out. I was just leaning back in the chair with this smirk on my face, telling him everything, and I mean everything. Mary Beth was looking at me, astonished. I felt like the more I told him, the better my chances were that he would figure me out. I told him about the moods, the anger, the fights, and work. I told him what I struggled with personally and family-wise. I told him about my issues at work and the problems my injury had caused. I also told him how I fought with retention issues and with trying to understand new information or changes in work tasks. I told him I always tried to avoid taking medicine because I was afraid it would make some deficits impossible for me to identify. Although that may be the point in taking the medicine, I was afraid the problem would come back even worse.

Mary Beth continued to stare at me as I poured everything out; sometimes she would laugh at the fact that I was "emptying out the closet." I recall smiling at the doctor when I was done with an "okay, now let's see if you can fix that" look. It felt great to talk with someone who might understand. I said what I had to. If I hid anything, I thought that would make the visit pointless.

The doctor smiled at what had taken place. The first thing he said was how impressed he was that ten years after the injury and with all that had gone on, I was sitting there realizing that I could no longer win this fight. He commented that realizing I could no longer fight was a positive sign, and one that very few would have the guts to admit so long after the injury. I appreciated that comment, though I think a sign of intelligence would have been taking the doctor's advice about ten years earlier. Dr. Kay said his research showed that the majority of brain injury survivors took their frustration with things they could control out on family.

It seemed my unwillingness to treat something that was never going away was hurting every part of my life. I decided I did not ever want to experience another year that bore any resemblance to the last ten. I had this *thing*, and there was nothing I could do about it. And no, I was not the same person I was on the morning of November 21, 1992; I was the person whose life dramatically changed at 12:10 a.m., November 22, 1992.

We talked for a long time, and tests were then conducted. Dr. Kay had me visually follow a pen and showed Mary Beth how my eyes would shake as they went from side to side. He explained that this was a sign of significant damage, which made its way into the portion of the brain that controls the eyes' muscles and nerves. I told him that when I was tired, my right leg dragged and I seemed to shut down. I explained that it felt like my memory went from the size of a school bus to the size of a two-seat sports car.

He recommended a drug that would stop the lows and highs. He explained that my emotions needed a ceiling and a floor. We talked about how that could change my life and, if it didn't, what the next step would be. I asked how long it would be before we recognized any changes. He said it would be a while, and I should start the medicine as soon as possible. I think the possibility that something could change for the better put a smile on my face.

The problem with seeing any doctor after a brain injury, whether it is two months after the injury or ten years after, is that they never knew you before the injury. The only version of you they have is the post-injury version. They may attribute every flaw or trait they find unusual to the injury. The first few years after my injury, all I did was try to prove I was fine. After my injury occurred, in my mind, I had to go back to work. I felt that if I did, it would prove to everyone that I was normal. I didn't want to admit to anything being wrong, and as I mentioned before, initially I didn't have the capacity to realize something was wrong. Of course, I think less is expected of us the first year or two; after that, explaining that a problem or deficit is attributable to a long-ago brain injury will not be considered credible, at least by those you work with or casually interact with. What the public can't see, the public cannot understand.

I wanted to stay and talk to the doctor for hours; I know for me it felt like heaven to talk with someone I assumed "gets it." The truth is, doctors do not comprehend what you are going through; they just understand it enough to hopefully provide you with tools to help offset what is missing. Eventually, I left and was given another date for follow-up.

When I left, I was so excited to take the *magic medicine*. The medicine prescribed was called Tegretol. I was so sick of the life I had come to know, from work to just being me. I hated every part of it. I had a renewed sense of optimism when I left and was excited to get home and show the kids what the happy, optimistic version of me looked like. They hadn't had the chance to see that side in quite a while.

Back to work the following day with another opportunity to experience a hallmark moment. You can never have enough of these special times. I was called into Ron's office to review why we failed to pick up the two banks during the *Toys for Tots* volunteer effort that had taken place two days earlier. He went off on me, shouting about how I was a horrible manager. I sat there, not really paying attention to anything except that my respect level for this individual was about as low as it could get, and I was determined to let whatever he said fade into the office walls. My visit to the hospital the day before and the chance that maybe my life was going to be better as a result was what I was thinking about. He was pacing back and forth behind his desk, and finally he finished his motivational speech and I was allowed to leave. As I put my hand on the doorknob, he said, "You're pathetic." I left my hand on the doorknob, still thinking about what the doctors had told me the day before, and slowly turned and looked at him. I smiled and shook my head, and then I left the office. I was making some progress just knowing that maybe better days were in front of me.

Where is reality TV when you need it? I know my ratings would have been off the charts. Imagine watching these past ten years on a big screen. I have to admit, I would have liked to have seen so much of what I don't recall or simply struggled to understand. Having a brain injury is a non-stop ride, and you can't get off. There are times you feel like you have control, and then there is the other ninety percent of the time. The best cure for a life with a brain injury, in my opinion, is simplicity and a little understanding. I have failed at my attempts to simplify my life and paid the price.

The next few weeks came and went, and I was expecting to feel a drastic change from the medicine, only to discover that it just didn't work that way. I made a trip back to the hospital to meet with Dr. Kay again, and as always, those trips were like going to see the great "Wizard of Oz" for me. The effects of the prescribed medicine were more apparent to those around me than to me. The effects were very small but significant to a point. Those around me noticed a calming effect. When I refer to those around me, of course, I am referring to my family. As always, the ones closest to you are the first to see the bad and the good. To the rest of the world, you are who you are when they encounter you. The feedback from my family was positive, and after a while I began to notice a reduction in the *downs* as well as a reduction in the *highs*. I began to notice situations where I may have now reacted in a positive fashion as opposed to a negative response. No medicine is a cure-all; you need to do your part as well. I needed to avoid trying to do too much. I needed to avoid stressful situations. Stressful situations for me were like pouring sand in a car's gas tank. I needed to choose my battles wisely. Never had a phrase fit so perfectly. I also needed to keep doing the things in life that made me happy, such as hobbies. The fact is, the more content I am with life, the better I react to everything and everyone.

I was always someone who needed to feel some sort of satisfaction from my work. Self-satisfaction was always important to me, but never as important as it was after my injury. In the early process of rehabilitation, it is amazing what gets you adulation. If you make it through the day without instructions, those close to you consider that a great day. I remember rehabilitation when the therapist would give me puzzles to put together. When I would complete the puzzle, they would pat me on the back and tell me how well I did. It made me feel like a dog that finally knocked on the door when it had to use the outdoor facilities. However, I would be lying if I said it didn't create a smile on my face. When the doctor would ask, "Brian, do you know what year this is?" and I answered correctly, that was something he considered a victory. The company that once gave me the opportunity to feel satisfaction from my job often no longer provided that chance. It was not UPS that took the feeling away from me; it was a few individuals under the company's roof that were responsible. Unfortunately, I just watched the clock and hoped for better days.

In 2003, I did something I thought I would never do. I went to school, sort of. One of the staff managers at my office who knew what had taken place the year before encouraged me to go to school. Due to his position, he was involved in the meetings regarding my disability leave and the efforts of my manager to remove me from the company. This gentleman brought me into his office and told me how to get enrolled in a college program and obtain my degree in a timely fashion. He told me that I should consider pursuing employment at one of our competitors or another company once I obtained my degree. He meant that in a supportive way, and told me that I had plenty to offer and my skills would be appreciated.

This college had a format that was perfect for someone with my deficits to get a degree. With this particular school, a recognized university under the company's education program, I could complete the majority of my classes over the Internet at a pace that was comfortable for me. I had to write papers for certain classes, but most of the assignments could be completed online. I was awarded credits for my management experience at UPS. With credits for my experience and a bit of determination, I finished within two years. What a great feeling. The irony was that if I hadn't suffered a traumatic brain injury, I likely would have never earned my college degree.

There was another unique experience in 2003, and the outcome of this event was exactly what I hoped it would be. I always wanted to visit the hospital in Milwaukee where I was transferred after my initial diagnosis. If you recall, I explained how I was the first on record to *escape* from the hospital's neuro-intensive care unit. I have no memory of being at this hospital, probably because I was in a coma for the majority of my stay.

I decided to take the two-hour drive. Upon arriving, I tried to imagine what it felt like for family members to pull up to this place knowing that my chances for survival were doubtful. I made my way inside and befriended one of the hospital employees. I explained what had happened and told him how much I would appreciate being shown the neuro-intensive care unit (NICU). He agreed to take me there, and off we went.

When we arrived in the NICU, he called the nurses over and introduced me. He told them I had been there ten years ago. From there I told them the circumstances and asked the nurses if there was a chance that one or some of them remembered me. Most replied that they did not work at the hospital at that time. In what seemed like a slow-motion moment, a nurse came up to me and hugged me as tightly as I believe she could. She said, "I absolutely remember you." She seemed almost ready to cry. She told me that it was rare that they ever had anyone return post-injury. From there she took my arm and brought me over to the bed I was in, and she told me how on those few occasions I was awake I always asked for Coca-Cola. I asked her about the great escape, and she remembered. The nurse laughed as she showed me the security doors I managed to get through, and then she described how they found me in puddle of blood in the bathroom. I thanked her for tolerating me and for the medical care they had given me.

That visit really meant a lot to me. I think part of me wanted to see if anyone remembered me, and if so, I wanted to show how far I had come. Yes, I was hoping something would trigger my memory, but no such luck. It was great that someone shared with me another part of my life that I will never remember.

At UPS we tend to have the same division manager for about three to five years, and then they move on to another location or department. Sometimes you are sorry to see them go, and sometimes you are glad to see them move on. I would say this move definitely went under the "glad to see him move on" category. Ron's transfer took place sometime near the end of 2003, and a new manager was brought in. We are going to call him Neil. Neil was a quiet, nice guy. He seemed to be trying to adjust to the position as well as the Chicago-land area. We got along just fine, and he was somewhat comical. Sometime during his tenure, I brought all my sales awards in as well as any other recognition I had received during the years 1996 to 1999. I brought those awards in to prompt my new manager to see me differently than how I was certain I had been described to him; I knew he was told I had suffered a brain injury. Neil would walk by and bow to my awards, which always made me laugh. Eventually, I brought those awards back home. I felt they got more mileage in my basement.

During the summer of 2005 Neil took me out to lunch for what is referred to at UPS as a *career discussion,* or, as I began to call it, *passed-over discussion.* I never had a desire to move up the corporate ladder. All I ever wanted was a job that I enjoyed. For me, what you get paid means nothing if you don't enjoy what you do. If you can or do have a job you actually like, I mean truly like, you win.

Neil and I had a general discussion regarding basic work issues, and much to my surprise, he asked me about my brain injury. That was a first, and it felt good that someone actually cared enough to ask. He wanted to know the changes or differences in me after the injury. I had been waiting and hoping for someone to ask me that question, and it was really nice to talk about it. Even more so, it was a relief that someone actually cared enough to ask. I think he heard about what had happened a few years earlier was trying to get me to open up about it.

When we were finished eating, Neil said, "I looked into your records, and it appears that you were doing quite well...and then your career went downhill." He was referring to a time after my injury. "Are you aware of who destroyed your career and why?"

"Yes, I am pretty sure I know who they were, and I am pretty sure I know why."

He then confirmed that those responsible for my career destruction had done an excellent job destroying it. "You basically have to start over," he said.

"That part I can't understand," I replied.

There really was no chance of *starting over* due to the barriers I would have had to overcome in order to be considered a contributor again. I knew my career was destroyed the day I sent my résumé out to everyone involved in sales in my region and not one person replied. They all knew me, or they thought they knew me. To follow that up, in 2002, when I returned from my three months off, I was told that I would never be allowed to return to sales.

We talked for quite a while, and he was very complimentary, and what took place with my career seemed to really bother him. It felt good to finally have someone who saw me as an individual who had skills and abilities, brain injury or not.

At the time I could not understand why he did something so extremely thoughtful, something he didn't have to do. I figured it out two days later when he resigned. He left a phone message with the company, and we never saw him again. I believe he did it to let me know that he didn't agree with the way I had been treated. Or maybe he just did it to be nice. I'm not sure where he is these days, but wherever you are, Neil, thank you.

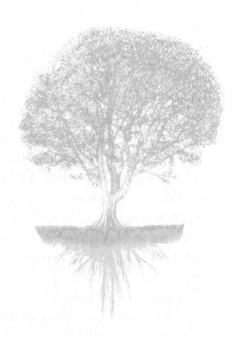

the invisible fight

As of right now, I am just trying to raise my children and manage my life as best I can. I continue to try to simplify my life and realize that I have a long way to go, but I'm making progress. I don't view my doctors as "Wizards of Oz" anymore. I realize they can only do so much, and I need to do the rest. I realize that I am truly lucky to have a life that most doctors were sure I would never have. I just need to stop and smell the roses more often.

I know my number-one enemy is stress. If there are hidden deficits from the injury, stress will find them and show them the way out. When I am alone, I over-think everything. Yet sometimes it actually helps to be alone. I review everything I am doing and try to figure out ways to be a better person. I cannot expect complete understanding regarding my life and what I struggle with nor can I change the fact that I have a TBI. I just try to deal with it and be thankful that I can do so many things as well as I do. I know my deficits could have been so much worse, and I realize how lucky I am. I hope to use my story as a tool for providing some understanding as to what it is people with brain injuries deal with on a daily basis.

I recently had a conversation with a co-worker, Joe, whom I have worked with since 1989. Joe knew me before my injury and was in the same office complex as I was in 2002 when the tornado hit my career. Joe told me that he always admired that no matter how bad things were for me, I never let on to any of my co-workers. Joe said that although he could tell at times I was dying internally, I always smiled and kept it to myself. When I walked out in 2002, Joe said that he and others in the office thought I was on vacation because I never said a word about it. Of course, they figured out that most vacations end after a week or two and assumed that something had gone wrong.

The truth was I was worried that I would be considered stupid if I admitted to not knowing something that others assumed I should know. When I was in a panic to learn something that I knew I should know, I always made sure I didn't ask the same person I'd asked the last time I needed help. That was my way of hiding that I was struggling.

Brain injuries make you feel trapped: you are made to feel that your injury has nothing to do with your shortfalls. The sad part is you are often treated unfairly, especially in the work environment, because others may believe that your deficits are exaggerated or are due to a perceived lack of intelligence. The truth is it takes a great deal of intelligence to create alternative approaches in order to compensate for your deficits. Your brain works in ways it never had before your twenty-one seconds. I have to remember that it's not what I have lost that counts; it's what I do with what I have left.

I still get those feelings of euphoria. I am sure they will be with me forever. I don't experience emotional changes at the same frequency I once did. I have developed the ability to manage or identify those changes somewhat better than I once was able to. I know that result-based activities trigger a great feeling or mood. I guess it has to do with being able to see a positive result to something I have done. For example, I can landscape for hours, and after I finish I can stare at the result for the longest time. One thing important to me and I would imagine is shared by most TBI survivors is recognition. These days, society seems to dwell more on what someone does wrong as opposed to recognizing what he or she may have done right.

I was asked recently if I believed I would have been treated differently if I had a physical deficiency to accompany the brain injury. The example this person used was, "If your paralysis never cleared up and you had to drag your leg or use a wheelchair, do you believe you would be treated differently?" I replied yes without hesitation. I have never been ashamed of the fact that I have a brain injury; I am proud of how far I have progressed. However, it really is unfortunate that these injuries are so misunderstood and quite complicated.

I still can't lock the car without the keys in my hand. I still do not carry a wallet. I try to minimize the things I have to keep track of or remember. I have tried to make daily tasks a routine. I leave myself messages in every way possible. To this day, I struggle with what feels like are versions of me that I don't care for or understand. I am doing better with that particular issue. Retention is still a major problem for me. Math scares me. I always said that if they want to really drive me out of my place of employment, put me in accounting.

Regardless of the unfortunate events that have taken place since my injury—and the sometimes realization that life may have been significantly different had I never suffered a TBI—I am proud of who I am and what I have accomplished. I am proud of my family, and I believe they are proud of me. I have had my share of bad days, but in my own way I came back more determined. There were times when walking away from situations that were pure pain would have been the preferred path; however, I didn't walk away. I try to keep a mental note of what I do that is good. I have to, because I tend to beat myself up over mistakes I have made and the way life sometimes makes me feel.

The version I know of me is an easygoing, "do anything for anyone" type of person. I enjoy making people laugh. I am credited with a great sense of humor. I love Mary Beth and my kids. My kids find me to be funny. My son Brian has told me that I am his best friend since the day he could speak, and at thirteen he still tells me that. Jim goes to school, works, works out, and spends time being a great kid. He laughs at things that I say, and he ignores me when I point out how much better his car would look if he introduced it to soap. Jenna is eleven and full of life. She is a great dancer and loves to be on stage. Jenna still makes me chase her before I can have a hug. Katie is currently finishing college and plans to move to Florida, but I am going to talk her out of it. Recently, she wrote a report for a college class, and the report was about my life as a TBI survivor and the challenges I faced. It was amazing how much she has seen and how much she tries to understand the whole brain injury mystery.

I thrive on keeping busy—not a "sitting in front of a computer" busy—but a physical busy. My perfect day would consist of waking at seven o'clock in the morning and washing the cars or changing the oil if it's due. After that, I hit the gym. From there my day would only get better if I fixed or built something.

All in all, it has been a strange and, at times, indescribable experience. And as much as I described events in my life that were sad due to the lack of understanding on behalf of those I have dealt with, I cannot say with any degree of certainty how I would have treated someone like me. I do hope I would have been more understanding. The whole point in writing this is to give those who have suffered a TBI a voice, and to provide understanding. There is no cure for brain injuries, and as long as there is life on earth, there will be brain injuries. The only steps in prevention, as well as recovery, are small steps. My wish is that in ten years someone else will write a book on brain injuries and it will be titled *Every 21 Minutes.*

I chose not to waste time worrying about the fact that I have a TBI. I have one and there is nothing I can do except cope with it. In regards to my recovery, I am proud of what I have accomplished. There were some difficult times, but those challenges were the costs I paid to recover my life; a life the experts said I would never regain. The truth is my life has been blessed since this injury as I have accomplished so much. This is not a book about how unfortunate my life has been since the injury; it is a story about how fortunate my life has been despite the injury. Yes, there are times I wish I could erase, but that is life. TBI or not, we all have times in our lives we wish we could erase or do over. I look forward to the future, and do all I can to make sure I enjoy it as best I can.

I would like anyone who has had a TBI to understand all the opportunities life holds for you, and that there is life after a TBI. I always viewed my injury as a speed bump, not a barrier, to what I want to accomplish. I do realize now there were times I tried to do too much, and I paid the price for it. Patience is really something you must learn when you have a TBI. Easier said than done, I know. The world of brain injuries is almost impossible to comprehend, for as much as we know about brain injuries, there is that much more we do not know. Yes, there are significant challenges following a TBI. However, always remember this: you are still capable of much more than you can ever imagine. Family support, proper treatment, and a positive belief in what you can accomplish are priceless when facing the challenges presented by traumatic brain injuries.

I pray that I've been a good dad and husband; I believe for the most part that I have. I hate that my children have had to see the ugly side of this injury. I spent a lot of time talking about the bad but I think my kids would tell you something different. I believe they would tell you I am a good person and a good father. I keep every Father's Day card they have given me. Here is what my son Jim wrote to me on Father's Day, 2007.

> *Dad,*
>
> *I'm so thankful to have a dad like you. You care about your family so much, and you would do anything for us. Thanks for always being there, and thanks for doing everything you can to make my life the best it can be. I look up to you in more ways than you would ever know. I dream to be half the man you are. I thank God every day that you survived that accident, because I don't know what I would have done without you. I thank God every day for having parents like you and Mom. Thanks for always knowing what was best for me and for letting me make my own decisions, even if sometimes you don't*

agree. I love you, Dad, and thank you for being the dad that you are.

Happy Father's Day.

Jim

Thank you, Jim.

photos

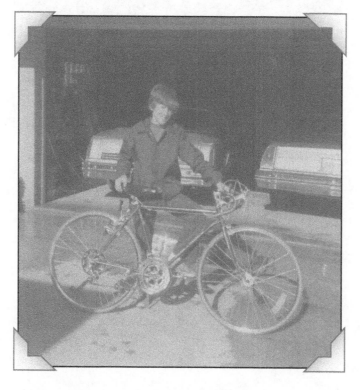

Every kids dream in the '70s was a Schwinn bicycle.
I still have this bike and it doesn't look any different.
Yes, the generator light still works.

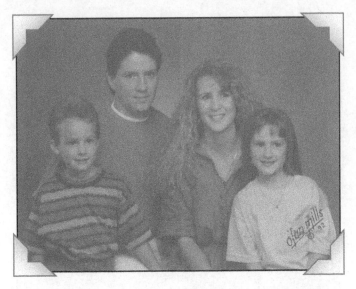

This photo was taken in October 1992, one month
prior to my brain injury.

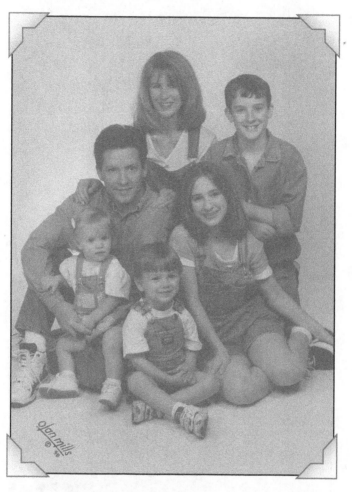

"Jeans fest 1998." Mary Beth and I with all four kids.

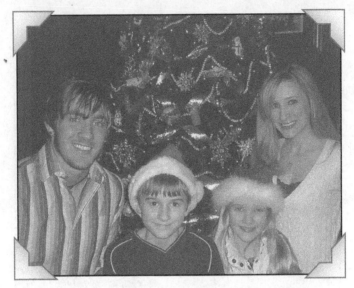

Christmas 2006. I love this picture.

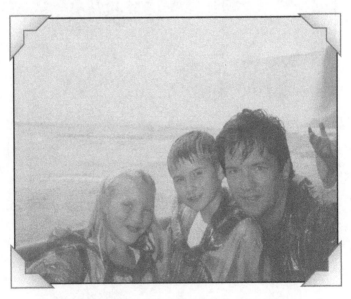

My favorite picture of the youngest two, Brian and
Jenna, with me at Niagara Falls.

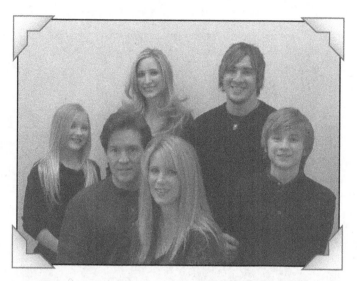

Taken at Christmas 2007. Looks like an '80s hair
band collided with the Brady Bunch.

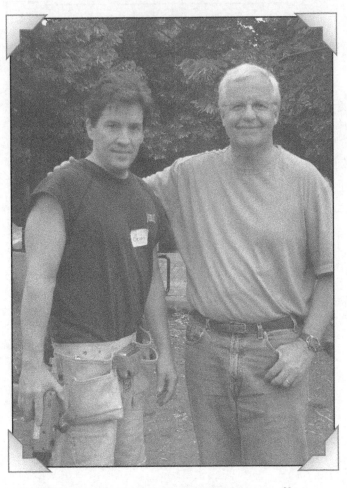

This photo was taken during a volunteer effort.
Along with other UPS employees, we assisted in
building a playground for disabled children. With
me is friend and co-worker Mike Ryan.

summary

As you read through my story, you may recall the deficits or affects of a brain injury that I have encountered—some were temporary, but others were permanent. Here are some statistics from the Brain Injury Association of Illinois regarding brain injuries.

Brain Injury Characteristics & Statistics:
Characteristics

Just as each individual is unique, so is each brain injury. Physical disabilities, impaired learning, and personality changes are common. Frequently reported problems include:

•• *Physical:* Speech, Hearing, Paralysis, Headaches, Vision, Seizure Disorder, Muscle Spasticity, Reduced Endurance.

•• *Cognitive Impairments:* Concentration, Attention, Perceptions, Planning, Communication, Writing Skills, Short-Term Memory, Long-Term Memory, Judgment, Sequencing, Reading Skills, Orientation.

Behavioral / Emotional Changes: Fatigue, Anxiety, Low Self-Esteem, Restlessness, Agitation, Mood Swings, Excessive Emotions, Depression, Sexual Dysfunction, Lack of Motivation, Inability to Cope, Self-Centeredness.

Statistics

• • 1.5 million Americans sustain a traumatic brain injury every year.

• • Each year 80,000 Americans experience the onset of long-term disability following TBI.

• • Among those who survive, 80,000 people per year must learn to cope with lifelong losses of function.

• • 5.3 Million Americans–two percent of the U.S. population currently live with disabilities resulting from a brain injury.

• • Motor vehicle accidents cause forty-four percent of brain injuries; falls, twenty-six percent; assaults and firearms, seventeen percent; sports and recreation and other, thirteen percent.

• • An estimated 200,000 children are hospitalized each year with brain trauma and 30,000 sustain permanent disabilities.

• • Every year in the U.S. 50,000 children sustain bicycle-related brain injuries; of those, over 400 die.

• • Males are twice as likely to sustain a brain injury than females, and young men between the ages of 15 and 24 have the highest rate of injury.

•• Every year, 50,000 Americans will die as a result of a traumatic brain injury.

•• "Last year, Veterans Affairs started screening all Iraq and Afghanistan war veterans who come in for clinical help. So far, 33,000 or 227,015, about 15 percent, have screened positive for mild brain injury since April 2007." (*New York Times*, Tuesday, August 26, 2007.)

Whatever the cause, a brain injury can, according to the Brain Injury Association of America, result in "an impairment of cognitive abilities or physical functioning. It can also result in the disturbance of behavioral or emotional functioning." Cognitive consequences can include memory loss, slowed ability to process information, trouble concentrating, organizational problems, poor judgment, and difficulty initiating activities, among others. Physical consequences can include seizures, muscle spasticity, fatigue, headaches, and balance problems, among others. Emotional/behavioral consequences can include depression, mood swings, anxiety, impulsivity, and agitation, among others.

Brain injury affects not only the individual, but the family, close friends, co-workers, and other social networks of the individual as well. Roles and relationships change; the financial ramifications may be extensive.

Mary Beth told me that I was satisfied with life prior to November 21, 1992. She said that I absolutely am different since that day. Her perspective is that I have been looking for something in my life that I may never find. I keep looking for that one piece of life that is going to make me feel like I did prior to that day in 1992. I guess I agree with that analysis. There is something missing, and I keep trying to fill that void. One thing I have always wanted to do was to tell my side of what life has been like since that day. I always believed I had the story that may just be interesting enough to make a difference.

I have this hope that my life will change for the good if my story gets told. Truth is, it would change because I know someone, somewhere, who is one of the 1.5 million a year who will suffer a TBI, may have a better life due to my writing this book. TBI survivors have a remarkable story, and I just wanted to be a voice for all of them.

One frustrating part of being a TBI survivor is the general perception by those who know you or work with you is that you *had* a brain injury. You see, you never *had* a brain injury; you will forever *have* a brain injury. These types of injuries never go away. On multiple occasions, eyes have rolled when something I was struggling with was tied to a brain injury that happened a few years ago. Sadly, some of those rolling eyes belonged to people who are close friends or family members. I hope what I have written will prevent anyone from ever rolling their eyes at the sometimes subtle and sometimes devastating effects of a brain injury. I hope companies who employ those of us with traumatic brain injuries take a look at how they work with us and realize all we are capable of. All we ask for are reasonable considerations.

I continue to make strides and take every opportunity to make a difference with traumatic brain injuries. In 2005, I was the topic of an article in a Chicago newspaper called "The Invisible Fight." This article was very well received, and the paper had multiple calls and letters regarding the article. The calls were from families who, unfortunately, had just had a family member suffer a TBI. I gave the newspaper the approval to provide the callers my e-mail address. From there I spoke with every single person who inquired. I also met with the injured. I made a difference; I am sure of it.

I try hard to be as good as I can at all I do. I still prefer doing things that display a result, something I can see. Whether it is something at work, building a deck, finishing a basement, it doesn't matter; the fact is, I love to look at something I built and know that I made it. Outside of work, I still run a hundred miles an hour, or at least my brain does. I spend a few days a week working out at the local health club, Body Tech. Some call it working out or exercising, I call it body maintenance.

I don't know what else I can say except thanks for reading my story. Unfortunately, too many people can associate with my story, and that is why I wrote it. For years I have kept so much to myself regarding what is locked inside. Writing this made me feel like I went from a whisper to a scream. I always wanted to open some eyes and minds with what still amazes me. Again, thanks to everyone who supported me through this journey, and special thanks to my family for giving me more tolerance than I deserve. There is one thing that I have to come to terms with: maybe I still see myself differently than others see me. Maybe the negative situations at work were due to something others may see that I don't. Granted, I try to view myself in the most positive light I can; however, maybe there are deficits that even I am not aware of. Regardless, not even that admission will ever justify what I experienced.

I hope I made a difference with this little walk through my personal history. I could continue to add to this story until the day I leave this earth, but I believe I have made my point.

I love music, always have, and there have been many days that music got me through. I always look for those with a purpose behind their songs. One of my recent favorites is a Jon Bon Jovi tune called "It's My Life." There is a line in that song that reads, "It's my life, it's now or never. I ain't gonna live forever. I just want to live while I'm alive…'cause it's my life."